Neuroendoscopy and Interventional Pain Medicine (*Volume 2*)

Endoscopy and Fetoscopy Techniques for the Brain and Neuroaxis

Edited by

Kai-Uwe Lewandrowski

Center for Advanced Spine Care of Southern Arizona and Surgical Institute of Tucson, Tucson, AZ, USA

William Omar Contreras López

*Clínica Foscal Internacional
Autopista Floridablanca - Girón, Km 7, Floridablanca
Santander, Colombia*

Jorge Felipe Ramírez León

*Fundación Universitaria Sanitas
Bogotá, D.C., Colombia*

Álvaro Dowling

*Orthopaedic Spine Surgeon, Director of Endoscopic Spine
Clinic Santiago, Chile*

&

Morgan P. Lorio

*Advanced Orthopedics, 499 East Central Parkway
Altamonte Springs, FL 32701, USA*

Assistant Editors

Hui-lin Yang

Professor & Chairman of Orthopedic Department
The First Affiliated Hospital of Soochow University
No. 899 Pinghai Road, Suzhou, China

Xifeng Zhang

Department of Orthopedics, Wangjing Hospital
China Academy of Chinese Medical Sciences, Beijing, China

&

Anthony T. Yeung

Desert Institute for Spine Care
Phoenix, AZ, USA

Neuroendoscopy and Interventional Pain Medicines

(Volume 2)

Endoscopy and Fetoscopy Techniques for the Brain and Neuroaxis

Editors: Kai-Uwe Lewandrowski, William Omar Contreras López,

Jorge Felipe Ramírez León, Álvaro Dowling & Morgan P. Lorio

ISBN (Online): 978-981-5274-49-3

ISBN (Print): 978-981-5274-50-9

ISBN (Paperback): 978-981-5274-51-6

need for a court order if at any point you breach any terms of this License Agreement. In no event will any delay or failure by Bentham Science Publishers in enforcing your compliance with this License Agreement constitute a waiver of any of its rights.

3. You acknowledge that you have read this License Agreement, and agree to be bound by its terms and conditions. To the extent that any other terms and conditions presented on any website of Bentham Science Publishers conflict with, or are inconsistent with, the terms and conditions set out in this License Agreement, you acknowledge that the terms and conditions set out in this License Agreement shall prevail.

Bentham Science Publishers Pte. Ltd.
80 Robinson Road #02-00
Singapore 068898
Singapore
Email: subscriptions@benthamscience.net

BENTHAM SCIENCE

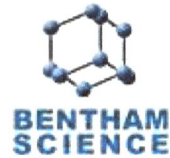

ENDORSEMENTS

SICCMI (Sociedad Interamericana Cirurgia de Columna Minimamente Invasiva)

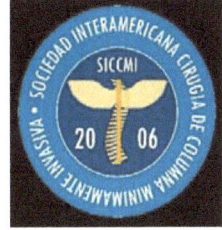

Founded in 2006, SICCMI aims to advance and mainstream minimally invasive spine surgery (MIS), aligning with the objectives of Neuroendoscopy & Interventional Pain Medicine. Our members have worked to implement MIS throughout South America, the Caribbean, Central America, and North America. Many of our key opinion leaders perform endoscopic surgery at the highest level and have contributed to this comprehensive multi-volume text. Four of the editors hold leadership positions within SICCMI. The table of contents is extensive, covering the cervical and lumbar spine and advanced technological applications. This book will serve as the core curriculum and course material for endoscopic spine surgery within SICCMI. It is my pleasure to endorse it on behalf of our society.

Alvaro Dowling

Past President of SICCMI

ISASS

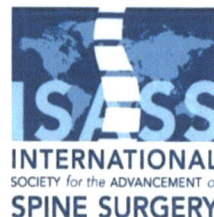

The origins of the International Society for the Advancement of Spine Surgery (ISASS), formerly known as The Spine Arthroplasty Society, can be traced back to its focus on motion preservation as an alternative approach to fusion. Over time, ISASS has remained dedicated to its overarching mission of serving as a worldwide hub for scientific exploration and education, centered around the needs of surgeons.

ISASS was established with the primary goal of creating an impartial platform where experts could openly discuss and tackle various aspects of both fundamental and clinical research related to motion preservation, stabilization, cutting-edge technologies, minimally invasive procedures, biologics, and other crucial subjects aimed at restoring and enhancing spinal motion and function. The society boasts a diverse and thriving global membership consisting of orthopedic and neurosurgery spine surgeons as well as scientists.

ISASS stands committed to pushing the boundaries of spinal techniques and procedures, including groundbreaking approaches like endoscopic spine surgery. A testament to this dedication is this text, Neuro-endoscopy, which serves as a reservoir of knowledge contributed by experts, resulting in a comprehensive and current reference text. This publication stands as a tangible example of our unwavering commitment to surgeon education and scientific advancement.

As representatives of ISASS, we take great pleasure in endorsing this all-encompassing text. It is a true reflection of our society's tireless pursuit of enhancing surgical education and promoting rigorous scientific exploration.

International Society for the Advancement of Spine – forging ahead on the path of progress.

Huilin-Lin Yang MD, PhD

ISASS Co-President, International 2023-2024

Morgan P. Lorio MD, FACS

Co-President Elect, USA 2024-2025

DR. KAI-UWE LEWANDROWSKI
AMCICO ENDORSEMENT
Neuroendoscopy and Interventional Pain Medicine

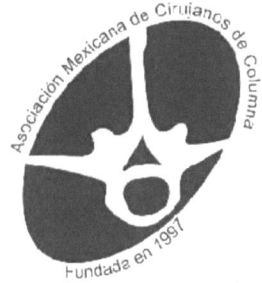

Asociación Mexicana de
Cirujanos de Columna A.C.

Dear Dr. Lewandrowski:

On behalf of the board of Asociación Mexicana de Cirujanos de Columna A.C (AMCICO) it´s an honor to endorse your upcoming groundbreaking text entitled *Neuroendoscopy and Interventional Pain Medicine*.

Your editors and authors highlighted the advancement and mainstreaming of minimally invasive surgery (MIS) for various topics in neurosurgery, spine surgery, and novel interventional pain management strategies involving the endoscopic technology platform. AMCICO members recently joined to discuss the implementation of MIS endoscopic surgery techniques in Mexico, where many of its key opinion leaders, some of whom have contributed to this outstanding text, perform endoscopic surgery at the highest level. The book content is exhaustive and comprehensive, encompassing cervical and lumbar spine topics with advanced technology applications. Moreover, your text highlights endoscopic surgery techniques of the cranium and skull base and, for the first time, describes the prenatal intra-uterine endoscopic repair of spina bifida. Neuroendoscopy and Interventional Pain Medicine will serve as AMCICO's core curriculum and course material for endoscopic surgery of the spine and neurological system. It is my pleasure to endorse it on behalf of AMCICO.

Again, we thank you for your valuable academic contribution and reiterate our disposition to assist with disseminating your outstanding text.

Sincerely

Dr. Eulalio Elizalde Martinez

President of AMCICO

Junta Directiva 2021 - 2023

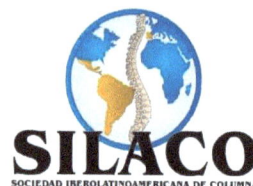

Dr. Jaime Moyano
Presidente

Dr. José Antonio
Soriano
1er Vicepresidente

Dr. Paulo Pereira
2do Vicepresidente

Dr. José Gabriel
Rugeles
Secretario

Dr. Álvaro Rocchietti
Tesorero

Dr. Hani Mhaidli
Presidente Anterior

Comisión Científica
Dr. Jorge Alves
Dr. Juan P. Bernasconi
Dr. Nicolás Galli
Dr. Mario
Herrera
Dr. Ratko Yurac
Dr. Juan José
Jara
Dr. Antonio Martín B.
Dr. Robert Meves

Comisión Fiscal
Dr. Eugenio Galilea
Dr. Alberto Diez
Ulloa
Dr. Luis Miguel Duchén
Dr. Roberto Muscia

SILACO (Sociedad Ibero Latinoamericana de Columna) had its beginnings in the meetings of the Scoliosis Research Society with the first Hispano-American Congress held in 1991 in Buenos Aires Argentina.

Since then, it has morphed into an organization that promotes the study of treatments and prevention of spinal conditions by bringing together spine care professionals from all subspecialties.

The scientific activities of our biannual Ibero-Latin American Congress are focused on the promotion of surgeon education to the highest academic standards via international relationships between members from the Americas, Spain and Portugal.

Neuroendoscopy and interventional Pain Management resembles such a collaborative effort where authors worldwide have come together to update the reader on the latest endoscopic spinal surgery techniques.

SILACO has incorporated Neuroendoscopy and interventional Pain Management into its core curriculum and plans on using it as course material for its continuing education courses.

It is my pleasure to endorse it on behalf of SILACO.

Dr. Jaime Moyano
President of SILACO

Editor SEOT Magazine
Ecuadorian Society of Orthopedics and Traumatology – SEOT

SOMEEC - Sociedad Mexicana de Endoscopia de Columna

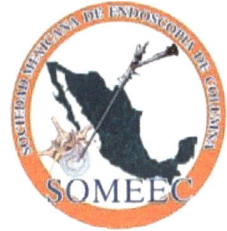

SOMEEC - Sociedad Mexicana de Endoscopia de Columna – is Mexico's prime organization uniting spine surgeons with diverse training backgrounds who have a fundamental interest in endoscopic surgery. SOMEEC organizes annual meetings where member surgeons and international faculty update each other on their latest clinical research to promote spine care via endoscopic spinal surgery techniques. Two of the senior lead editors of Neuroendoscopy & Interventional Pain Medicine have been active international supporters of SOMEEC. I am pleased to endorse their latest three-volume reference text, Neuroendoscopy & Interventional Pain Medicine which will become an integral centerpiece of SOMEEC's continuing medical education programs.

Enrique Saldívar Farrera

President of the Sociedad Mexicana de Endoscopia de Columna

Roberto Cantu, Jr. MD

Vice President of the Sociedad Mexicana de Endoscopia de Columna

Academia Nacional de Medicina de Colombia

The Academia Nacional de Medicina de Colombia recognizes the high academic and scientific value of the comprehensive three-volume text Neuroendoscopy & Interventional Pain Medicine. developed by leading figures in the field—including our esteemed members of our Academy, Dr. Kai-Uwe Lewandrowski, William Omar Contreras, and Dr. Jorge Felipe Ramirez—represents a significant advancement in minimally invasive spinal surgery. It will undoubtedly serve as an essential resource for both current and future spine specialists, greatly enhancing clinical practice and patient outcomes.

Gabriel Carrasquilla MD, DrPH, MPH, MSc
President, Academia Nacional de Medicina de Colombia

Asociación Colombiana de Neurocirugía (ACNCx)

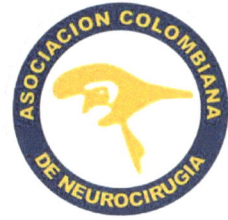

The Asociación Colombiana de Neurocirugía (ACNCx) is a non-profit, private legal entity dedicated to promoting the scientific and ethical development of neurosurgery in Colombia. Established in 1962, ACNCx is committed to advancing professional responsibility, continuous improvement, and the highest standards of patient care. ACNCx operates with a democratic structure, upholding principles of solidarity, unity, and participation. Our association is deeply involved in the education and advancement of neurosurgical practices, including innovative procedures such as prenatal endoscopic repair and endoscopic interventions for the brain, neuroaxis, and spine.

It is with great pleasure that I endorse Neuroendoscopy & Interventional Pain Medicine on behalf of ACNCx. This book highlights the groundbreaking work of Colombian authors and serves as a valuable resource for our members and the broader neurosurgical community.

Best Regards,

Alberto Dau Acosta

President

Colombian Association of Neurosurgery

International Society for Minimally Invasive Spine Surgery (ISMISS)

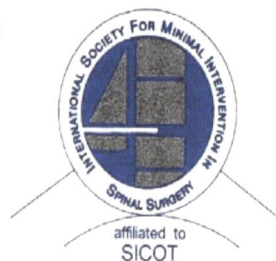

affiliated to
SICOT

The International Society for Minimal Intervention in Spine Surgery (ISMISS) brings together spine surgeons from all over the world united by the constant strive for advances in minimally invasive techniques. Since its conception in 1988 on the occasion of the GIEDA-Bruxelles meeting, international coordination of educational, instructional, and scientific exchanges in minimally invasive spine surgery has been the highest priority for prior and current directories.

As the newly elected president of ISMISS, it is my great pleasure to endorse Neuroendoscopy & Interventional Pain Medicine as an extraordinary textbook of up-to-date collaborative expertise in endoscopic techniques of the spine and neuroaxis. I am convinced that it will contribute significantly to the educational process of future spine specialists.

Prof. Dr. Joachim Oertel

President ISMISS

Chinese Orthopaedic Association (COA)

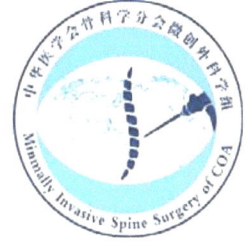

Chinese Orthopaedic Association (COA), a specialty society within Chinese Medical Association, was founded in 1980. It aims to promote scientific exchange, provide orthopaedic education, and improve patient care. COA is the largest and most influential orthopaedic society in China, equivalent to AAOS in the US. Its annual meetings attract about 15,000-32000 attendees, including world-class experts, presidents of international orthopaedic societies, and leaders from national orthopaedic associations.

In line with its mission to foster global discussions and enhance surgeon education, it is my pleasure as Chairman of the COA MISS Society to endorse Neuroendoscopy & Interventional Pain Medicine. This comprehensive text, created by an international team of editors and contributors, including many from China, provides an expert update on the latest endoscopic spinal surgery techniques.

I am confident that this book will become an essential part of any reputable spine surgeon society's core curriculum and serve as valuable course material for continuing education programs. It is my honor to support Neuroendoscopy & Interventional Pain Medicine on behalf of the COA MISS Society.

Huilin Yang

Professor Huilin Yang

Chairman of COA MISS Society

Japanese Minimally Invasive Spine Surgery Society (JASMISS)

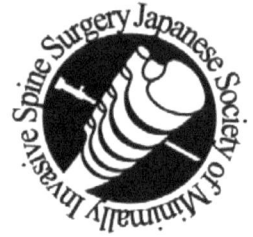

As JASMISS president I am interested in discussing advancements in surgical techniques, and collaborate on clinical trials. Through these initiatives, we continue to foster a collaborative environment that supports the continuous improvement and adoption of minimally invasive techniques in spine surgery.

This dedication to excellence is evident in Neuroendoscopy & Interventional Pain Medicine, which features numerous contributions from Asian authors showcasing their groundbreaking work. It is my pleasure to endorse Neuroendoscopy & Interventional Pain Medicine.

Professor Koichi Sairyo, MD, PhD

President of the Japanese Society of Minimally Invasive Spine Surgery (JASMISS)

Tokushima University, Japan.

Korean Research Society of Endoscopic Spine Surgery (KOSESS)

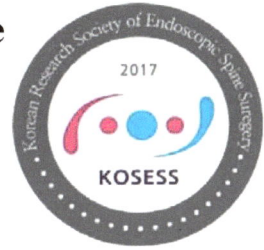

Founded in 2017, the Korean Research Society of Endoscopic Spine Surgery (KOSESS) aims to unite endoscopic spine surgeons in the Republic of Korea to advance the subspecialty through high-quality clinical research. This dedication to excellence is evident in Neuroendoscopy & Interventional Pain Medicine, which features numerous contributions from Korean authors showcasing their groundbreaking work.

It is my pleasure to endorse Neuroendoscopy & Interventional Pain Medicine on behalf of KOSESS.

Chang-il Ju M.D.,Ph.D.
President of KOSESS
Professor
Department of Neurosurgery
Chosun University Hospital
Gwangju, Korea
H.P. 010-3666-4100

Sociedade Brasileira de Coluna (SBC)

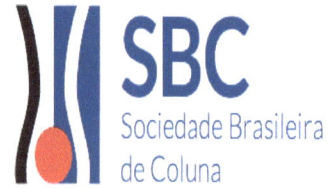

Founded on October 12, 1994, the Brazilian Spine Society (Sociedade Brasileira de Coluna - SBC) is a scientific, non-profit organization dedicated to advancing spine surgery through basic research and clinical studies in Orthopedics and Neurosurgery. SBC is committed to the accreditation and continued education of spine surgeons in Brazil, providing its members with access to the latest scientific evidence and technological advancements in spine care. Through its monthly publication, Columna, and various online courses, including an Introduction to Endoscopy, SBC strives to keep its members at the forefront of the field.

The editors of Neuroendoscopy & Interventional Pain Medicine have created a comprehensive reference text that is essential to SBC's core curriculum for teaching endoscopy of the spine and neuroaxis. This book presents validated clinical protocols for the endoscopic treatment of cervical and lumbar spine conditions, backed by peer-reviewed articles from its contributors.

It is my pleasure to endorse Neuroendoscopy & Interventional Pain Medicine on behalf of the Brazilian Spine Society. This work will undoubtedly play a crucial role in educating the next generation of spine surgeons in Brazil.

Dr. Robert Meves

President of SBC

Sociedad Colombiana De Cirurgia Ortopedia Y Traumatología(SCCOT)

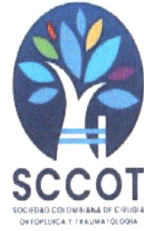

The Sociedad Colombiana de Cirugía Ortopedia y Traumatología (SCCOT) is a non-profit, autonomous, scientific organization committed to enhancing spine care and surgery for orthopaedic and neurosurgeons, as well as other healthcare professionals in Colombia. Established to foster collaboration and innovation, SCCOT unites specialists with diverse scientific interests and expertise. Our goal is to promote continuous professional development and education, ensuring our members are well-versed in the latest advancements in spinal care.

With great enthusiasm, on behalf of SCCOT, endorse the three-volume book series Neuroendoscopy & Interventional Pain Management. This text is of significant interest to SCCOT due to its advanced technological applications and comprehensive discussion of validated clinical protocols for endoscopic spinal surgery and neuroaxis interventions.

The editors of this landmark series are esteemed leaders in minimally invasive spine surgery. Their combined expertise and dedication to advancing the field are evident throughout the volumes, making this series an invaluable resource for spine surgeons and related professionals.

Neuroendoscopy & Interventional Pain Management will serve as a cornerstone for SCCOT's continuing medical education programs. The extensive table of contents covers crucial topics related to the cervical and lumbar spine, as well as the latest technological advancements. This series will undoubtedly become a vital part of our educational initiatives, equipping our members with the knowledge and tools to excel in their practice.

I am honored to endorse this significant work on behalf of SCCOT. The dedication and expertise of the editors have produced a reference text that will shape the future of spine surgery and improve patient care worldwide.

Dr. William Arbeláez Arbeláez

President Sociedad Colombiana de Cirugía Ortopedia y Traumatología (SCCOT)

Sociedad Latinoamericana de Ortopedia y Traumatologia (SLAOT) / Latin American Society of Orthopaedics and Traumatology

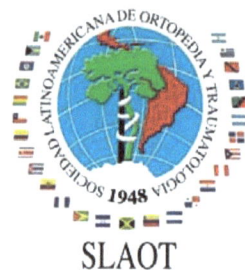

SLAOT

The Sociedad Latinoamericana de Ortopedia y Traumatologia (SLAOT) is a non-profit, autonomous, scientific organization dedicated to orthopaedic surgeons and care professionals. SLAOT unites experts with diverse scientific interests, promoting continuous professional development and education at the highest level.

Neuroendoscopy& Interventional Pain Managementis highly relevant to SLAOT due to its exemplary use of advanced technology and detailed discussion of validated clinical endoscopic spinal surgery protocols. It is my pleasure to endorse this comprehensive text on behalf of SLAOT.

Dr. Victor Naula

President of SLAOT FEDERACION

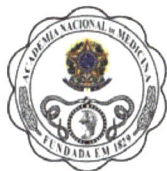

Academia Nacional de Medicina

Av. General Justo, 365 – 7º andar - Centro - Rio de Janeiro - RJ

www.anm.org.br

**Diretoria
Biênio 2024-2025**

Presidente
Eliete Bouskela

1º Vice-Presidente
Antonio Egidio Nardi

2º Vice-Presidente
Ronaldo Damião

Secretário Geral
Omar Lupi da Rosa Santos

1º Secretário
Mônica Roberto Gadelha

2º Secretário
José Hermógenes Rocco Suassuna

Tesoureiro
Henrique Murad

1º Tesoureiro
Rossano Kepler Alvim Fiorelli

Orador
Natalino Salgado Filho

Diretor de Biblioteca
Jayme Brandão de Marsillac

Diretor de Arquivo
Miguel Carlos Riella

Diretor de Museu
Arno von Buettner Ristow

Presidente da Secção de Medicina
José Galvão-Alves

Presidente da Secção de Cirurgia
José de Jesus Peixoto Camargo

**Presidente da Secção de Ciências
Aplicadas à Medicina**
Walter Araújo Zin

Rio de Janeiro, august 22, 2024

Commendation of *Neuroendoscopy & Interventional Pain Medicine*

The Academia Nacional de Medicina de Brazil remains steadfast in its commitment to advancing medical knowledge, fostering education, and upholding the highest standards in patient care. It is with great honor that we commend Dr. Kai-Uwe Lewandrowski, one of our esteemed members, and his team of leading experts for their exemplary work in producing *Neuroendoscopy & Interventional Pain Medicine*. This timely three-volume text significantly contributes to the field of minimally invasive spinal surgery and stands as an invaluable resource for current and future spine specialists, enhancing clinical practice and improving patient outcomes.

Eliete Bouskela
Presidente

Academia
Nacional de
Medicina

Sociedad Colombiana De Columna (SOCCOL)

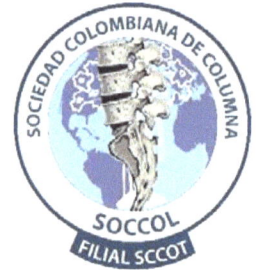

The Sociedad Colombiana de Columna (SOCCOL) is a non-profit, autonomous, scientific organization dedicated to advancing spine care and surgery among orthopaedic and neurosurgeons, as well as other care professionals in Colombia. Founded to foster collaboration and innovation, SOCCOL brings together experts with diverse scientific interests and backgrounds. Our mission is to promote continuous professional development and education, ensuring our members stay at the forefront of the latest advancements in spinal care.

It is with great enthusiasm that I, on behalf of SOCCOL, endorse the three-volume book series Neuroendoscopy & Interventional Pain Management. This comprehensive text is particularly significant to SOCCOL due to its exemplary use of cutting-edge technology and detailed discussion of validated clinical endoscopic surgery protocols for the spine and neuroaxis.

The editors of this landmark series are distinguished leaders in minimally invasive spine surgery. Their collective expertise and dedication to advancing the field are evident throughout the volumes, making this series an invaluable resource for spine surgeons and affiliated professionals.

Dr. Kai-Uwe Lewandrowski, a pioneer in endoscopic spine surgery, has greatly contributed to the development and refinement of minimally invasive techniques. Drs. Jorge Ramírez, Alvaro Dowling, and William Contreras, esteemed members of the Latin American spine surgery community, have played key roles in promoting these advanced surgical practices across the region. Dr. Anthony Yeung and Dr. Xifeng Zhang, world-renowned experts, have extensively published on endoscopic spine surgery and interventional pain management, further solidifying the series' credibility. Drs. Morgan Lorio and Huilin Yang are visionary minimally invasive spine surgeons who have been instrumental in prompting policy changes at national and international levels.

Neuroendoscopy & Interventional Pain Management serves as a cornerstone for SOCCOL's continuing medical education programs. The comprehensive table of contents covers topics related to the cervical and lumbar spine, as well as advanced technological applications. This series will undoubtedly become an integral part of our educational initiatives, providing our members with the knowledge and tools necessary to excel in their practice.

I am honored to endorse this significant work on behalf of SOCCOL. The dedication and expertise of the editors have resulted in a reference text that will shape the future of spine surgery and enhance the quality of care for patients worldwide.

Dr. Connie Bedoya

President of SOCIEDAD COLOMBIANA DE COLUMNA (SOCCOL)

Sociedade Brasileira de Neurocirurgia (SBN)

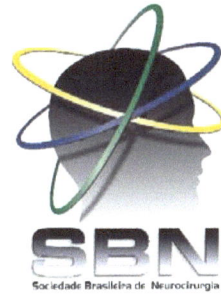

The Brazilian Society of Neurosurgery (SBN), established in 1957 in Brussels and affiliated with the WFNS since 1959, has been instrumental in shaping neurosurgical education and practice in Brazil. Notably, SBN was one of the first societies in the country to require examinations for the title of master, beginning in 1972. SBN continues to encourage high standards in neurosurgery through continuous education and international collaboration and is deeply involved in shaping the curriculum and standards for neurosurgical residency programs, ensuring that both fundamental and clinical research are integral parts of neurosurgical training.

In line with our commitment to excellence, I am proud to endorse Neuroendoscopy & Interventional Pain Medicine on behalf of BSN. This textbook, crafted by global leaders in minimally invasive spine surgery, serves as an invaluable resource that will enhance the education and practice of future neurosurgical specialists.

Dr. Wuilker Knoner Campos

President,

Sociedade Brasileira de Neurocirurgia

Brazilian Society of Neurosurgery (SBN)

CONTENTS

PREFACE

Welcome to Neuroendoscopy and Interventional Pain Medicine, Vol. 2: Endoscopy and Fetoscopy Techniques for the Brain and Neuroaxis. This volume centers on sophisticated techniques and critical considerations in the rapidly developing field of advanced neuroendoscopy of the brain, anterior and posterior skull base, and spinal cord for pain, tumors, and seizures, mainly focusing on advanced intracranial, intradural, and fetoscopic procedures. It brings together the collective expertise of renowned specialists, offering an invaluable resource for clinicians and researchers dedicated to enhancing patient care through innovative surgical approaches.

The book begins with a comprehensive overview of the State-of-the-Art direct endoscopic visualization of the brain and neuroaxis, highlighting the latest advancements in imaging and visualization technologies that have revolutionized neurosurgical practices. One chapter sets the foundation for understanding the complex anatomy and pathological conditions that neuroendoscopy addresses. Trigeminal tractotomies and nucleotomies explore targeted endoscopic interventions for trigeminal neuralgia and other intractable facial pain syndromes. This chapter aims to improve outcomes for patients suffering from these debilitating conditions by providing detailed procedural insights. The endonasal endoscopic approaches to the sellar region and the anterior fossa chapter discuss minimally invasive techniques for accessing and treating pathologies in these critical regions. The authors present step-by-step methods and highlight the benefits of these approaches in reducing patient morbidity. Understanding the pathophysiology of myelomeningocele & modern surgical treatment is crucial for developing effective management strategies for this congenital condition. This chapter thoroughly examines the underlying mechanisms and contemporary fetoscopy options available to clinicians. Building on this knowledge, fetoscopy techniques for myelomeningocele outline the prenatal interventions that can be performed to mitigate the effects of myelomeningocele. The authors share cutting-edge fetoscopic techniques that hope for improved outcomes in affected fetuses. For the treatment of cancer pain, microendoscopic intradural cordotomy offers a minimally invasive option. This chapter details this approach's procedural aspects and efficacy, which targets the pain pathways within the spinal cord to provide relief for patients with intractable pain. The endoscopic anatomy of the transcallosal hemispherectomy based on a cadaver study with advanced 3D modeling provides a unique perspective on the anatomical intricacies of this procedure. Using advanced 3D modeling, the authors offer valuable insights into the endoscopic anatomy, facilitating better surgical planning and execution. Outcomes of endoscopic treatment for early correction of craniosynostosis in children present the benefits and results of early intervention for this congenital skull deformity. This chapter underscores timely surgical correction's importance in promoting normal brain development and growth. The chapter on autonomic dysreflexia with hypertension following durotomy-related intradural spread of irrigation fluid and air during routine spinal endoscopy addresses a severe but rare complication of spinal endoscopy. The authors discuss the pathophysiology, recognition, and management of autonomic dysreflexia to enhance patient safety. Finally, a commonly overlooked issue during thoracic spinal endoscopy is given credence in this volume's final chapter, highlighting the importance of preoperative identification of the Adamkiewicz System. A thorough preoperative workup is needed to avoid catastrophic complications during thoracic spinal endoscopy. By identifying Adamkiewicz's artery system, surgeons can better navigate the thoracic spine and reduce the risk of spinal cord ischemia.

Each chapter in this volume has been meticulously selected to reflect contemporary trends and innovations in neuroendoscopy of the brain, anterior and posterior fossa, brain stem, and relevant interventional pain management procedures. By addressing the need for safer, more efficient, and cost-effective solutions, this book aims to meet the demands of patients, healthcare providers, and policymakers. The editors hope that Vol. 2 of Neuroendoscopy and Interventional Pain Medicine: Intra- and Extradural Endoscopy & Fetoscopy Techniques of the Brain and Neuroaxis serves as an indispensable resource for clinicians and researchers committed to advancing the field and improving patient care.

Kai-Uwe Lewandrowski
Center for Advanced Spine Care of Southern Arizona and Surgical
Institute of Tucson
Tucson, AZ, USA

William Omar Contreras López
Clínica Foscal Internacional
Autopista Floridablanca - Girón, Km 7, Floridablanca
Santander, Colombia

Jorge Felipe Ramírez León
Fundación Universitaria Sanitas
Bogotá, D.C., Colombia

Álvaro Dowling
Orthopaedic Spine Surgeon, Director of Endoscopic Spine Clinic
Santiago, Chile

Morgan P. Lorio
Advanced Orthopedics, 499 East Central Parkway
Altamonte Springs, FL 32701, USA

Assistant Editors

Hui-lin Yang
Professor & Chairman of Orthopedic Department
The First Affiliated Hospital of Soochow University
No. 899 Pinghai Road, Suzhou, China

Xifeng Zhang
Department of Orthopedics, Wangjing Hospital
China Academy of Chinese Medical Sciences, Beijing, China

&

Anthony T. Yeung
Desert Institute for Spine Care
Phoenix, AZ, USA

List of Contributors

Alberto Di Somma	Division of Neurosurgery, Department of Neurosciences, Reproductive and Odontostomatological Sciences, Università degli Studi di Napoli Federico II, Napoles, Italy
Alberto G. Prats	Laboratory of Surgical Neuroanatomy, Faculty of Medicine, Universidad de Barcelona, Barcelona, Spain
Anthony Yeung	Desert Institute for Spine Care, Phoenix, AZ, USA
Benedikt Burkhardt	Wirbelsäulenzentrum / Spine Center – WSC, Hirslanden Klinik Zürich, Witellikerstrasse 408032 Zurich, Switzerland
Claudio Rivas-Palacios	Department of Pediatric Neurosurgery. Napoleon Franco Pareja Children's Hospital (Child's House), Cartagena, Colombia Center of Biomedical Research (CIB), Faculty of Medicine, University of Cartagena, Cartagena, Colombia
Cristóbal Abello Munárriz	Centro Médico CEDIUL, CEDIFETAL, Barranquilla, Colombia
Edgar G. Ordóñez-Rubiano	Department of Neurosurgery, Hospital de San José – Fundación Universitaria de Ciencias de la Salud, Los Mártires, Bogotá, Cundinamarca, Colombia
Elvira Puello F.	Department of Pediatric Neurosurgery. Napoleon Franco Pareja Children's Hospital (Child's House), Cartagena, Colombia Faculty of Medicine, University El Sinu, Cartagena, Colombia
Ernesto Luis Carvallo Cruz	Department Chief of Neurological Surgery, Hospital Vargas de Caracas, Caracas 1010, Venezuela
Erich Talamoni Fonoff	Division of Functional Neurosurgery of Institute of Psychiatry, Department of Neurology, University of São Paulo Medical School, São Paulo, Br
Ezequiel García-Ballestas	Department of Pediatric Neurosurgery. Napoleon Franco Pareja Children's Hospital (Child's House), Cartagena, Colombia Center of Biomedical Research (CIB), Faculty of Medicine, University of Cartagena, Cartagena, Colombia Latinamerican Council of Neurocritical Care (CLaNI), Bogota, Colombia
Guido Parra Anaya	Departamento de Ginecología y Obstetricia, División de Medicina Maternofetal, Clínica General del Norte, Barranquilla, Colombia
Javier G. Patiño-Gómez	Department of Neurosurgery, Hospital de San José – Fundación Universitaria de Ciencias de la Salud, Los Mártires, Bogotá, Cundinamarca, Colombia
Jezid Miranda Quintero	Departamento de Ginecología, Facultad de Medicina, Grupo de Investigación en Cuidado Intensivo y Obstetricia (GRICIO), Universidad de Cartagena, Cartagena de Indias, Colombia
Jordi Rumià	Department of Neurosurgery, Hospital Clinic, Faculty of Medicine, Universidad de Barcelona, Barcelona, Spain
Jose Pineda	Laboratory of Surgical Neuroanatomy, Faculty of Medicine, Universidad de Barcelona, Barcelona, Spain

Joachim Oertel	Universitätsklinikum des Saarlandes, Neurochirurgische Klinik, Gebäude 90, Kirrberger Straße, 66421 Homburg (Saar), Germany
Jorge Felipe Ramírez León	Minimally Invasive Spine Center, Bogotá, D.C., Colombia Reina Sofía Clinic, Bogotá, D.C., Colombia Fundación Universitaria Sanitas, Bogotá, D.C., Colombia
Juan David Hernandez	Sociedad Colombiana de Anestesiología, Departamento Anestesiología, Clínica General del Norte, Barranquilla, Colombia
Kai-Uwe Lewandrowski	Center for Advanced Spine Care of Southern Arizona and Surgical Institute of Tucson, Tucson, AZ, USA Departmemt of Orthopaedics, Fundación Universitaria Sanitas, Bogotá, D.C., Colombia Department of Neurosurgery in the Video-Endoscopic Postgraduate Program at the Universidade Federal do Estado do Rio de Janeiro - UNIRIO, Rio de Janeiro, Brazil
Leonardo Domínguez	Department of Pediatric Neurosurgery. Napoleon Franco Pareja Children's Hospital (Child's House), Cartagena, Colombia Department of Neurosurgery, University of Cartagena, Cartagena, Colombia
Marco Moscatelli	Clinica NeuroLife, Natal, RN, Brazil
Mario M. Barbosa	Trauma and Emergency Epidemiology Research Group, University of Valle, Cali, Colombia
María Andrea Escobar	Faculty of Medicine, Rafael Nuñez University, Cartagena, Colombia Department of Arts and Humanities, International University of Valencia, Valencia, Spain
Miguel Parra Saavedra	Departamento de Ginecología y Obstetricia, División de Medicina Maternofetal, Clínica General del Norte, Barranquilla, Colombia Universidad Simón Bolívar, Barranquilla, Colombia
Morgan P. Lorio	Advanced Orthopedics, 499 East Central Parkway, Altamonte Springs, FL 32701, USA
Nadin J. Abdalá-Vargas	Department of Neurosurgery, Hospital de San José – Fundación Universitaria de Ciencias de la Salud, Los Mártires, Bogotá, Cundinamarca, Colombia
Nicolás Rincón Arias	Department of Neurosurgery, Hospital de San José – Fundación Universitaria de Ciencias de la Salud, Los Mártires, Bogotá, Cundinamarca, Colombia
Oscar Zorro	Department of Neurosurgery, Hospital de San José – Fundación Universitaria de Ciencias de la Salud, Los Mártires, Bogotá, Cundinamarca, Colombia
Paulo Sérgio Teixeira de Carvalho	Pain and Spine Minimally Invasive Surgery Service at Gaffre e Guinle University Hospital, Rio de Janeiro, Brazil
Pedro Roldán	Department of Neurosurgery, Hospital Clinic, Faculty of Medicine, Universidad de Barcelona, Barcelona, Spain
Peter Winkler	Paracelsus Medical University of Salzburg, Strubergasse 21, 5020 Salzburg, Austria

René O. Varela   Department of Neurosurgery, Universidad del Valle, Instituto Neurológico del Pacífico, Valle del Cauca, Colombia

Roth A.A. Vargas   Department of Neurosurgery, Foundation Hospital Centro Médico Campinas, Campinas SP, Brazil

Stefan Landgraeber   Universitätsdes Saarlandes, Klinik für Neurochirurgie, Kirrberger Straße 100, 66421 Homburg, Germany

William Omar Contreras López   Clínica Foscal Internacional, Autopista Floridablanca - Girón, Km 7, Floridablanca, Santander, Colombia

State-of-the-Art in Direct Endoscopic Visualization of the Brain and Neuroaxis

Ernesto Luis Carvallo Cruz[1], **William Omar Contreras López**[2,*], **Kai-Uwe Lewandrowski**[3,4,5], **Stefan Landgraeber**[6], **Jorge Felipe Ramírez León**[7,8,9], **Peter Winkler**[10], **Benedikt Burkhardt**[11] and **Joachim Oertel**[12]

[1] *Department Chief of Neurological Surgery, Hospital Vargas de Caracas, Caracas 1010, Venezuela*

[2] *Clínica Foscal Internacional, Autopista Floridablanca - Girón, Km 7, Floridablanca, Santander, Colombia*

[3] *Center for Advanced Spine Care of Southern Arizona and Surgical Institute of Tucson, Tucson, AZ, USA*

[4] *Departmemt of Orthopaedics, Fundación Universitaria Sanitas, Bogotá, D.C., Colombia*

[5] *Department of Neurosurgery in the Video-Endoscopic Postgraduate Program at the Universidade Federal do Estado do Rio de Janeiro - UNIRIO, Rio de Janeiro, Brazil*

[6] *Universitätsdes Saarlandes, Klinik für Neurochirurgie, Kirrberger Straße 100, 66421 Homburg, Germany*

[7] *Minimally Invasive Spine Center. Bogotá, D.C., Colombia*

[8] *Reina Sofía Clinic. Bogotá, D.C., Colombia*

[9] *Fundación Universitaria Sanitas. Bogotá, D.C., Colombia*

[10] *Paracelsus Medical University of Salzburg, Strubergasse 21, 5020 Salzburg, Austria*

[11] *Wirbelsäulenzentrum / Spine Center – WSC, Hirslanden Klinik Zürich, Witellikerstrasse 408032 Zurich, Switzerland*

[12] *Universitätsklinikum des Saarlandes, Neurochirurgische Klinik, Gebäude 90, Kirrberger Straße, 66421 Homburg (Saar), Germany*

Abstract: Over the past two decades, the endoscopic endonasal approach has significantly expanded the armamentarium of minimally invasive skull base surgery. Initially developed for the treatment of pituitary adenomas, endoscopic endonasal skull base surgery (EESBS) has found increasing utility in managing a broad spectrum of skull base pathologies. Its application extends from the midline, encompassing the crista galli process to the occipitocervical junction, and laterally to the parasellar areas and petroclival apex. In recent years, there has been a notable shift from the exclusive use of endoscopic technology in endonasal pituitary surgery to other neuroendoscopic

* **Corresponding author William Omar Contreras López:** Clínica Foscal Internacional, Autopista Floridablanca - Girón, Km 7, Floridablanca, Santander, Colombia; Tel: +573112957003; E-mail: wyllcon@gmail.com

procedures. This chapter aims to provide the reader with an up-to-date overview of clinical trials on endoscopic neurosurgery of the skull base, brain, and neuroaxis. Through a comprehensive review of the state-of-the-art published peer-reviewed literature, the authors strive to offer a concise summary of the current concepts in this rapidly advancing field.

Keywords: Brain, Direct visualization, Endoscopic surgery, Neuroaxis, Skull base.

INTRODUCTION

Technological advancements have played a pivotal role in the expansion of endoscopic visualization in the field of brain and neuroaxis. This innovative tool has emerged as a transformative technique, granting neurosurgeons unparalleled access during surgical procedures. Direct endoscopic visualization necessitates specialized endoscopes equipped with high-definition cameras and illumination systems. When combined with three-dimensional imaging systems, these high-definition cameras offer neurosurgeons an immersive and highly detailed view of the surgical field. This superior visualization facilitates the identification of critical structures and improves spatial orientation. Moreover, this technique provides a minimally invasive alternative to traditional open surgery, mitigating the risks associated with extensive tissue disruption while enhancing surgical precision and patient outcomes.

The boundaries of transnasal endoscopic surgery in the pituitary fossa have been surpassed, and its applications now extend from the midline, spanning from the crista galli process to the occipitocervical junction. It extends laterally to the parasellar areas and petroclival apex in the posterior skull base. The ability to directly visualize pathological structures, assess lesion extent, and precisely target treatment sites has made neuroendoscopy a competitive alternative to traditional open surgery for treating brain tumors, vascular malformations, hydrocephalus, and other conditions affecting the brain and neuroaxis. Furthermore, the applications of endoscopic surgery extend beyond conventional neurosurgery, finding utility in diagnostic biopsies, intracranial pressure monitoring, and cerebrospinal fluid management.

The advantages of direct endoscopic visualization are manifold. By utilizing smaller incisions or natural orifices, this technique minimizes tissue trauma and reduces the risk of complications such as infection, bleeding, and scarring. Additionally, endoscopes' magnification and illumination capabilities enable surgeons to visualize structures with enhanced clarity and precision, thereby promoting optimal decision-making during surgery. Moreover, this technology contributes well to integrating augmented reality and virtual reality platforms, further improving surgical planning and intraoperative navigation, thereby fostering safer and more efficient procedures. Furthermore, the minimally invasive nature of neuroendoscopy often results in shorter hospital stays, faster recovery times, and improved patient satisfaction. In this chapter, the authors aim to provide an up-to-date overview of clinical trials on endoscopic neurosurgery of the skull base, brain, and neuroaxis.

Historical Perspectives

Since the dawn of the 20th century, endoscopic neurosurgical modalities have evolved significantly. Hermann Schloffer initiated the transsphenoidal access in 1906, innovatively accessing a pituitary neoplasm via the sphenoid bone. L'Espinasse, in 1910, employed a cystoscope for choroid plexus fulguration in two infants, heralding success in one [1]. Walter Dandy's 1922 endeavor for a choroid plexectomy found no success [2]; however, 1923 saw Mixter's landmark achievement with an endoscopic third ventriculostomy (ETV) using a urethroscope on a pediatric patient [3]. Scarff later introduced a state-of-the-art endoscope in 1935, playing a pivotal role in addressing hydrocephalus arising from benign aqueductal stenosis or periaqueductal masses [1, 4].

The paradigm shifted with Nulsen and Spitz's introduction of ventricular cerebrospinal fluid (CSF) shunting in 1952 [5]. Nevertheless, 1959 marked the ushering in of modern endoscopy through the rod-lens system developed by Harold Hopkins. By 1963, Gerard Guiot made noteworthy strides with a fiberoptic endoscopic transnasal transsphenoidal intervention. Yet, the operating microscope retained its supremacy, especially in skull base surgeries [5].

With the emergence of coupled-charge devices from Bell Laboratories in 1969, video-endoscopy found its footing, and was subsequently honed by Karl Storz. The subsequent decade observed an ETV renaissance for obstructive hydrocephalus, propelled by enhanced endoscopic visualization. In 1978, Vries delineated the ETV's potential using cutting-edge fiberoptic instruments [6]. Thereafter, Jones *et al.* highlighted evolving shunt-free success trajectories, peaking at 61% in a pool of 103 patients by 1994 [7] [8], with contemporary rates oscillating between 80% to 95% [1, 4 - 8]. In a further pioneering leap, 1992 saw Roger Jankowski *et al.* reporting the first endonasal pituitary excision via endoscopy [9], followed by Ricardo Carrau and Hae-Dong Jho's substantial series in 1997, encompassing 50 patients [10].

The Standards

Neuroendoscopy has evolved to encompass a plethora of conditions beyond traditional ventricular interventions. Now, its application extends to address intracranial cysts, intraventricular neoplasms, hypothalamic hamartomas, cranial base neoplasms, craniosynostosis, certain spine pathologies, specific hydrocephalus subtypes, among others. Modern neuroendoscopic suites, boasting high-definition endoscopic technologies, have exponentially enhanced surgical visualization and ergonomic efficiency, allowing seamless collaboration amongst multiple surgeons. In the following, the authors attempt to briefly touch on some of the current neuroendoscopic surgery standards without claiming complete description of the many protocol advances currently in various stages of clinical investigation in the fast moving field of neuroendoscopy.

Endoscopy in Hydrocephalus Management

Endoscopic third ventriculostomy (ETV) stands as the premier intervention for obstructive hydrocephalus, particularly in the context of aqueductal stenosis, with efficacy rates surpassing 60%. Additionally, ETV proves instrumental in managing hydrocephalus secondary to tectal plate lesions [1, 11]. Factors such as the hydrocephalus etiology and patient age play a pivotal role in ETV's success. While infants, especially those presenting with congenital hydrocephalus or myelomeningocele, may pose challenges, efficacy rates in older children and adolescents often eclipse 70% [12]. In instances of midline posterior fossa tumors precipitating acute hydrocephalus, a preoperative ETV can be contemplated, positioning it as a reliable substitute to shunt placement postoperatively [12]. Moreover, endoscopic techniques, including septostomy, septum pellucidotomy, fenestration of compartmentalized ventricles, and aqueductoplasty, address intricate hydrocephalus manifestations. Procedures like foraminoplasty at the foramina of Monro and Magendie, as well as endoscopic fourth ventriculostomy, further expand its applicability [1, 13, 14].

Endoscopic Management of Cysts and Intraventricular Neoplasms

Endoscopic techniques are indispensable in cyst fenestration, tumor biopsies, excisions, and biopsies of metastatic disease. Specifically, hydrocephalus stemming from suprasellar or quadrigeminal arachnoid cysts can be adeptly addressed via endoscopic fenestration. Given that a significant proportion of patients with intraventricular cysts or tumors manifest concomitant hydrocephalus, the endoscopic approach proffers the dual benefit of CSF redirection and neoplastic management [15, 16]. Current-day endoscopic tumor biopsies have gained substantial traction, boasting an impressive success rate (>90%) coupled with minimal risks (<3.5%) [17]. The methodology has rendered invaluable insights in the context of germ cell tumors, insidious hypothalamic/optic pathway gliomas, and Langerhans cell histiocytosis. For colloid cysts or pedunculated ependymal tumors, endoscopic excision stands as a viable strategy, barring instances of expansive cysts where risks associated with venous injury at the foramen of Monro elevate [14] (Fig. **1**).

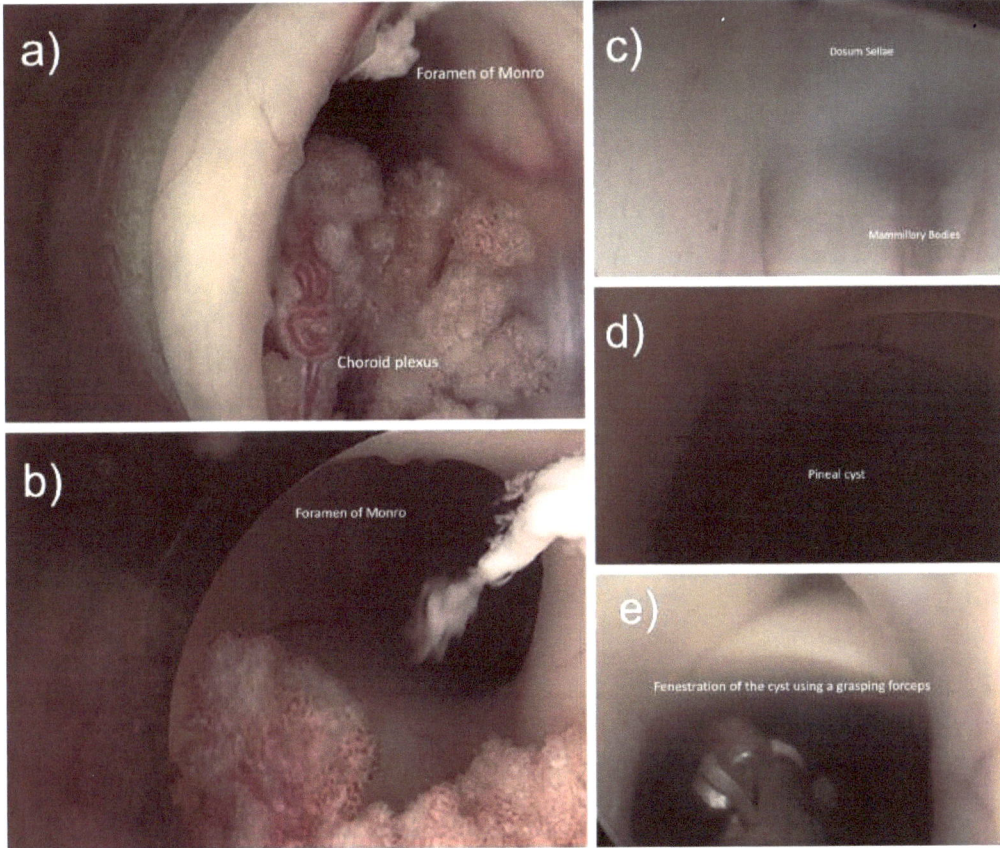

Fig. (1). (**a**) Shown are endoscopic views of the right lateral ventricle with choroid plexus and foramen of Monro, (**b**) view into the foramen of Monro, (**c**) view onto the floor of the third ventricle, (**d**) view onto the pineal cyst, (**d**) fenestration of the cyst.

Endoscopic techniques may proficiently address craniopharyngiomas, hypothalamic chiasmatic astrocytomas, as well as suprasellar and pineal germ cell tumors. However, complete resection of solid neoplasms is occasionally constrained due to instrumental limitations and hemostatic challenges. The efficacy of these endoscopic tumor excisions is contingent upon tumor dimensions, consistency, and vascularity [14, 17]. Additionally, endoscopic modalities have been effectively employed in the management of extraventricular arachnoid cysts located at sites such as the Sylvian and interhemispheric fissures and the posterior fossa, enabling safe fenestration from the cyst into the adjacent subarachnoid space [15].

Endoscopic-aided Craniosynostosis Management

Jimenez and associates were at the forefront of minimally invasive interventions for craniosynostosis [18, 19]. Optimal intervention using endoscopy-assisted craniosynostosis surgery (EACS) is feasible within the first six months of life, augmented with subsequent helmet molding therapy; the paradigm age being three months. This intervention, employing standard instruments alongside a 0° endoscope, is akin to those used in endoscopic facelift procedures. Concurrent blood aspiration is conducted using a dedicated aspirator. Documented outcomes highlight minimal complications and impressive success rates [19]. An ensuing section provides an in-depth discussion on EACS. For scaphocephaly, a meticulous craniectomy extending from anterior to posterior fontanelle is executed, and the removed bony strip measures roughly 4-5 cm in width and about 11 cm in length. Ancillary osteotomies can be orchestrated posterior to the coronal suture and anterior to the lambdoid sutures. Outcomes from this approach have been commendable, with only a fraction (9% of 139 subjects) necessitating transfusion [14, 18, 19]. Post-procedure, pediatric patients are advised a helmet for roughly ten months, initiated three weeks post-operatively, with vigilance towards potential dermal complications, which are infrequent.

Endoscopic Interventions for Hypothalamic Hamartoma (HH)

Hypothalamic Hamartomas (HHs), a cohort of uncommon non-malignant congenital anomalies emanating from the inferior hypothalamus, manifest with distinct clinical syndromes such as gelastic seizures, early-onset puberty, and cognitive disturbances. Aside from those presenting with premature puberty, surgical intervention is typically warranted. Depending on HH typology, varied or combined therapeutic strategies are employed. For expansive HHs, transcallosal craniotomies are favored, while smaller lesions are amenable to gamma knife surgery or stereotactic radiofrequency thermocoagulation. Endeavors involving endoscopic resection coupled with stereotactic navigation have been piloted for smaller HHs, albeit achieving only partial resections [20]. Owing to the typical ventricular dimensions in these patients, navigational aid is often indispensable [20]. Contemporary literature posits that endoscopic disconnection of HHs potentially surpasses other techniques in safety and efficacy.

Advancements in Neuroendoscopic Spinal Procedures

Over recent decades, there has been a marked ascendance in the adoption of neuroendoscopic techniques for managing both intra- and extradural spinal anomalies. The endoscopic fenestration of intradural arachnoid cysts has been streamlined, whereas the previously favored dissection of septations within multiloculated syringomyelia cavities during the 1990s yielded mediocre clinical and radiographic outcomes [21]. In modern minimally invasive spinal interventions, the neuroendoscope has carved out a pivotal niche. Its repertoire has burgeoned to incorporate diverse procedures like thoracoscopic sympathectomy [22], discectomies [23 - 28], lumbar laminotomies [29], anterior spinal reconstructive strategies [30 - 33], excisions of neoplasms [34, 35] and cystic formations [36 - 39]. The prevalence of endoscopic discectomy in the thoracic [40 - 44] and lumbar spine [45 - 48] has surged. While epiduroscopy has been employed in the treatment epidural fibrosis post-spinal interventions [49 - 52], its definitive efficaciousness warrants continued investigative scrutiny.

Intraparenchymal Neuroendoscopic Approaches

Endoscopic advancements, marked by enhanced illumination and visualization, have capacitated surgical endeavors within the brain parenchyma [17, 53]. The marriage of a keyhole craniotomy paradigm [54] with judiciously chosen trajectories facilitates endoscopic access to intraparenchymal lesions in conjunction with navigation [36]. The instrumentation, inclusive of suction apparatus, tumor forceps, microscissors, and coagulative implements, is introduced through a dedicated sheath. Impeccable intraoperative irrigation and drainage are imperative to ensure a lucid endoscopic vista. Resection goals—whether intralesional or excisional—hinge on the tumor's characteristics. While the scope of these endoscopic interventions is evolving, their current applicability extends to pathologies such as cavernous angiomas, cerebellar infarctions, intraparenchymal hematomas, and cerebral abscesses [14]. The endoscopic modality, celebrated for its precision and safety, harbors potential for broader indications for the treatment of intraparenchymal lesions [14].

Neuroendoscopic Augmentation in Microsurgical Interventions

Neurosurgeons are increasingly inclined towards leveraging neuroendoscopy in concert with traditional skull base microsurgical techniques. The endoscope, complementing the microscope's robust capabilities, provides unparalleled access to intricate recesses, minimizing the need for undue retraction and meticulous skull base access. Though the microscope remains the principal tool in endoscope-augmented microsurgery due to its unparalleled image integrity, endoscopic strategies are currently reserved for trained surgeons in specialized institutions. The endoscope excels in elucidating bony or dural detail and intricate neurovascular configurations. While typically manipulated freehand for inspection, it can also be anchored to a stabilizing apparatus, facilitating bimanual dissection and proffering the surgeon unhindered bilateral manual dexterity [14, 55]. This synergistic methodology has manifested its prowess in diverse skull base surgeries—including tumor resections (*e.g.*, pituitary tumors, craniopharyngiomas, acoustic neuromas, and epidermoids), aneurysm occlusions, and trigeminal microvascular decompressions [14].

Endoscopic Innovations in Skull Base Surgery

The advent of neuroendoscopy has transformed the treatments for skull base neoplasms. Carrau *et al.* (1996) were pioneers in documenting their endeavors with endonasal transsphenoidal hypophysectomy [55], a legacy which was later expanded upon by de Divitiis *et al.* (1997) to encompass diverse sellar and parasellar pathologies [56]. Presently, the bilateral endonasal endoscopic stratagem facilitates comprehensive visualization from the anterior skull base's crista galli to the C2 vertebra. Notably, the endoscopic endonasal paradigm has showcased commendable efficacy and reduced morbidity in resecting pathologies such as pituitary adenomas and craniopharyngiomas. The choice of this modality for sellar or suprasellar lesions hinges on their extent, with supradiaphragmatic variants managed endonasally and suprasellar pre-chiasmatic infundibular abnormalities addressed via the trans-tuberculum-transplant sphenoidal technique [14].

Moreover, endoscopy has become instrumental in managing CSF rhinorrhea of diverse etiologies. Endoscopic interventions enable meticulous cranio-sinonasal space delineation, fostering multilayered reconstructions. While small bony defects are typically addressed with autologous fat or fascia accompanied by tissue sealant, sizable openings, especially with pronounced intraoperative CSF leaks, mandate a multi-tiered closure, amalgamating autologous fat grafts, fascia lata, bony buttresses, and tissue sealants. In scenarios of severe skull base abnormalities, the incorporation of a gasket seal closure becomes indispensable [14].

Endoscopic Skull Base Surgery (ESBS) has ascended to be a gold standard for several afflictions including pituitary macroadenomas, cerebrospinal fluid rhinorrhea, and anterior skull base meningiomas, among others. Beyond neurosurgery, otolaryngologists have embraced ESBS for a spectrum of pathologies, ranging from olfactory neuroblastoma (notably Kadish A and B types) to recurrent nasopharyngeal malignancies. The past triad of decades has witnessed a meteoric rise in ESBS adoption, with a significant proportion of nonfunctional pituitary adenomas now addressed via this modality. A meticulous survey revealed an overwhelming majority of skull base surgeons, encompassing both neurosurgeons and otolaryngologists, incorporating ESBS techniques in their armamentarium [57].

Advances in Transnasal Neuroendoscopic Interventions

Transnasal neuroendoscopic procedures epitomize minimally invasive endeavors targeting profound intracranial entities via the nasal conduit. An exhaustive analysis of extant literature has elucidated the multifaceted clinical applications, outcomes, merits, and limitations of this methodology. This exploration spanned a gamut of neurosurgical anomalies, from pituitary tumors to ventricular discrepancies. Accumulated evidence underscores the efficacy and safety profile of transnasal neuroendoscopic interventions, extolling their reduced morbidity, expedited recovery, and improved patient satisfaction [55], while ensuring surgical outcomes on par, if not surpassing, conventional methodologies [58]. Nonetheless, mastery of this technique presents a formidable learning curve, with its share of potential pitfalls. To nurture proficiency amongst the next generation, the lead author has instituted biannual cadaveric workshops in the postgraduate curriculum, focusing on hands-on exposure to this nuanced technique (Fig. **2**).

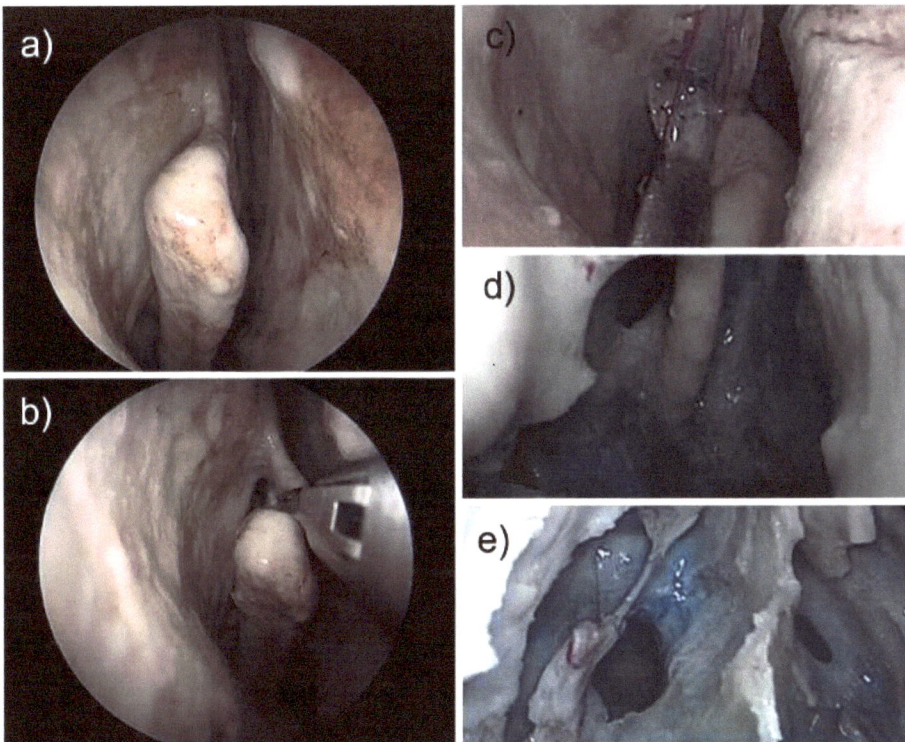

Fig. (2). Endoscopic views taking during the first author's biannual cadaver training course organized for residents of his postgraduate training program: **a**) view of medial cornet at lateral view, **b**) septum medial, **c**) cutting the medial cornet, **d**) cutting middle turbine and creating flap, **d**) vomer and ostium sphenoidal, **e**) keel of vomer, ostium bilateral sphenoids.

A comprehensive review of PubMed, MEDLINE, and Embase was undertaken to search for studies released exclusively between 2020 and 2023. The research strategy hinged on an amalgamation of specific terminologies: "transnasal neuroendoscopy," "transnasal endoscopic surgery," "skull base lesions," "pituitary tumors," "ventricular abnormalities," and "hydrocephalus." We centered our focus on investigations elaborating on clinical outcomes, surgical modalities, complications, and juxtapositions between transnasal neuroendoscopy and conventional open techniques. Literature spanning animal-based research, isolated case narrations, and non-anglophone compositions were systematically sidestepped. The task of data curation and integrity evaluation was spearheaded by a duo of independent examiners, anchoring their approach on the established PRISMA criteria. The preliminary exploration surfaced 20 manuscripts [59 - 78], of which a curated subset of 11 were deemed pertinent for this compendium [60 - 67, 76 - 78]. These chosen treatises spanned an array of neurosurgical anomalies, including but not limited to pituitary tumors and ventricular deviations. Overarchingly, the synthesized findings spotlighted the efficacy of transnasal neuroendoscopic interventions, often rivaling or eclipsing their traditional counterparts. Paramount benefits of this avant-garde technique encompass diminished post-operative challenges, expedited patient recovery, aesthetic enhancements, and heightened patient gratification.

In relation to pituitary neoplasms, transnasal neuroendoscopic intervention permits meticulous tumor excision, consistently achieving comprehensive resection and hormonal stabilization. When confronting skull base anomalies, this modality affords secure and efficient access to difficult-to-reach locales such as parasellar zones, clival malignancies, and the anterior cranial base, accompanied by minimal complications and augmented postoperative quality of life metrics (Fig. 3). A significant portion of the referenced studies are retrospective, casting doubt on their methodological rigor when juxtaposing endoscopic endonasal procedures against traditional microsurgical trans-sphenoidal techniques. Expert evaluations suggest potential superiority of the endoscopic route for certain pituitary adenomas, particularly in terms of total resection efficacy and an ostensibly smoother postoperative recovery. Beyond pituitary adenomas situated intra- and suprasellar, EESBS appears promising for lesions encroaching on the cavernous sinus, Meckel's cave, and clival regions. Within the domain of ventricular irregularities, the technique has excelled in endoscopic third ventriculostomies (ETV) and cyst fenestrations, diminishing shunt dependencies and their subsequent complications. In addressing hydrocephalus, this method presents a less invasive counterpart to conventional shunt interventions. However, the prevailing concern remains cerebrospinal fluid leakages, representing the principal shortcoming of this strategy.

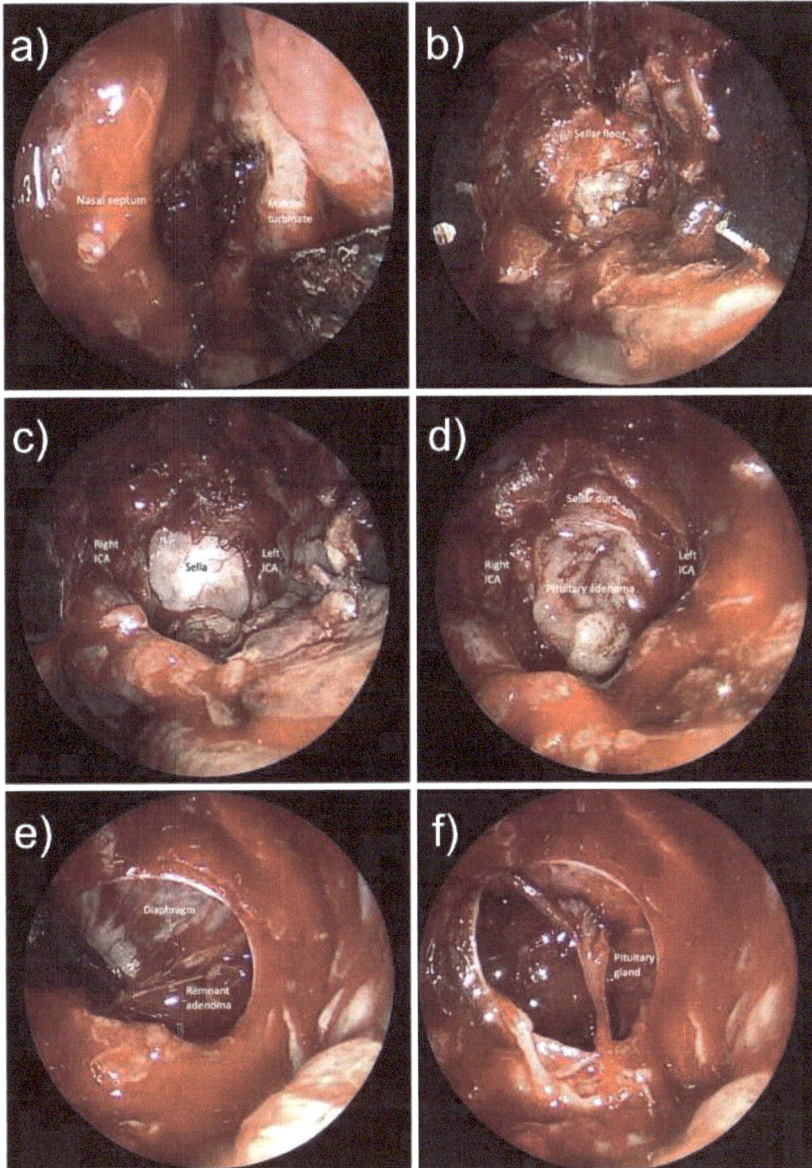

Fig. (3). Endoscopic views during transnasal surgery for pituitary adenoma show: **a)** left sided mononostril approach to sphenoid sinus floor, **b)** view of sellar floor after removal of spheonid sinus floor, **c)** anatomy of sphenoid sinus after opening of sellar floor with dura intact, **d)** phase of adenoma removal after opening of tumor capsule, **e)** view at diaphragm with some small remnants of adenoma tissue, **f)** identification of gland tissue after adenoma removal.

Martinez-Perez *et al.* furnished a meticulous review on the viability and safety of endoscopic endonasal clipping (EEC) as an alternative conduit to address centrally located intracranial aneurysms [58]. They undertook a comprehensive exploration of PubMed and Cochrane repositories, adhering to PRISMA guidelines, focusing on intracranial aneurysms subjected to EEC up until 2019. Data from these studies, encompassing clinical manifestations, radiographic data, and outcomes, were meticulously analyzed. Their review unveiled 9 studies, accounting for 27 patients (8 males, 19 females) harboring 35 aneurysms. Out of these, four aneurysms remained unaddressed by EEC, with two necessitating adjunctive measures, reflecting an overall treatment efficacy of 86%. Adverse events were noted in 26% of patients, with cerebrospinal fluid leakage (18%) and ischemic events (15%) being predominant. Interestingly, posterior circulation aneurysms demonstrated a higher complication propensity than their anterior counterparts (62.5% vs. 10.5%). Moreover, ischemic challenges were pronounced in 50% of posterior circulation anomalies. While EEC holds promise, it's also linked to considerable risks, with observed complication rates surpassing those of conventional open or endovascular interventions. Despite the allure of transnasal neuroendoscopic procedures, with their merits of decreased morbidity, expedited recovery, superior aesthetic outcomes, and elevated patient contentment, prevailing data advocates for transcranial clipping and endovascular occlusion as the gold standards in intracranial aneurysm management.

Technical Aspects

Optimal image quality in neuroendoscopy hinges on several imaging attributes, including illuminance, brightness, and resolution. Illuminance quantifies the light intensity distributed over a specific surface [58]. Contemporary endoscopes predominantly employ xenon light sources due to their superior illuminance and faithful color rendition. Nonetheless, these high-intensity bulbs introduce potential thermal hazards to tissues. As an alternative, light-emitting diode (LED) sources have been introduced, presenting minimized thermal injury risks. Brightness, a function of both illuminance and the inverse square of distance, dictates the luminance perceived by an observer and, by extension, the endoscope's sensor [58]. In endoscopic skull base surgery (ESBS), strategic modulation of brightness is pivotal. Enhancing brightness, by either augmenting illuminance or reducing the endoscope's distance to the target, must be judiciously executed to evade thermal injuries.

Commercial endoscopes present in varying resolutions: high definition (1280 × 720 pixels), full HD (1920 × 1080 pixels), and ultra-HD or 4K (3840 × 2160 pixels) [79]. Such granularity proves invaluable for discerning anatomical structures at the necessary level of detail. To optimize visibility within constrained spaces, digital zoom capabilities have been integrated, albeit with the trade-off of a narrowed field of view relative to optical zoom [79]. Factors such as viewing distance and monitor size influence the discerned resolution. Within ESBS, preferred viewing distances oscillate between 80-120 cm, though they can span 99-152 cm. Ultra-HD configurations might even entail a maximum distance of 152 cm with monitors exceeding 101.6 cm. Concomitantly, larger monitors are typically paired with elevated resolution systems [80]. Operational space and the digital footprint of high-resolution systems, given their voluminous data files, bear considerations for both surgical functionality and data logistics.

Three-dimensional (3D) endoscopy, a burgeoning technology, offers surgeons a stereoscopic view that augments depth perception [81]. Although such stereoscopic visualization has been trialed in operating microscopes, its universal adoption remains stifled by occasional side effects: nausea, visual strain, or migraines. Notably, mastering 3D visualization demands acclimation, especially as hand-eye coordination deviates from traditional 2D endoscopy. The salient advantage of 3D endoscopy, however, lies in its heightened depth field, achieved through dynamic camera motion and the tactile feedback from surgical tools navigating the operative site. While promising, further exploration of 3D endoscopy is essential to ascertain its optimal application parameters for maximum safety and efficacy.

Upcoming Developments

Technological progress has catalyzed advancements in neuroendoscopic surgical protocols. The evolution of optical technologies, cameras, and surgical tools has significantly expanded their clinical applicability in neurosurgery. Recent innovations, such as miniaturized multiport endoscopes and integration of robotics and navigation systems, have transformed the surgical treatment of several neural axis disorders, as detailed in subsequent chapters.

Neuronavigation systems, employing either optical image guidance or electromagnetic tracking, leverage computer modeling and preoperative images to enhance surgical precision by correlating intraoperative coordinates with imaging data [82, 83]. Moreover, these systems are increasingly utilized in virtual reality platforms, like the Dextroscope and NeuroTouch Endo, for neurosurgical training, offering tactile feedback, trainee performance tracking, and feedback mechanisms [84]. The computer-generated reconstruction of the patient is then referenced to determine the current location of calibrated instruments relative to preoperative imaging [82, 83]. Outside the operating room, adaptations of these systems have been integrated into virtual reality platforms for neurosurgical training [85]. For ESBS, these platforms include the Dextroscope (Volume Interactions, Bracco Group, Milan, Italy) and NeuroTouch Endo (National Research Council of Canada, Ottawa, ON, Canada). These virtual reality platforms offer trainees haptic feedback during part-task training and scenario simulations, promoting the development of operative skills [85]. The advantages of virtual reality-based training platforms extend to their potential for tracking trainee progress and providing feedback on trainee development and training program curricula.

Augmented reality (AR) overlays critical anatomical outlines on endoscopic imagery, amalgamating personalized data with endoscopic views [83, 85]. Originating from 1980s operative microscopes, AR now enables surgeons to simultaneously view endoscopic and neuronavigation monitors [86], thereby enhancing intraoperative orientation [87] and reducing neurovascular injury potential. Modern tools, integrated with neuronavigation functionalities, streamline the surgical process while enhancing ergonomics and dexterity [88]. However, the limitations of neuronavigation, especially with magnetic-based systems and patient registration in ESBS, warrant consideration [89]. The advancements in augmented reality and its increasing integration into neurosurgical training and practice underscore the growing importance of neuronavigation-based technologies. Specific augmented reality training models have been developed for ESBS [90]. These training models allow trainees to gain exposure to various skull base pathologies before performing surgery on patients. Synthetic tissue models, such as the UpSurgeOn system (UpSurgeOn SRL, Assago, Italy), incorporate augmented reality to enable anatomical exploration beyond what is possible with the naked eye [91]. However, this technology is still in its early stages and requires extensive investigation.

Intraoperative Imaging is another area of active clinical research. For example, fluorescence agents have been utilized in endoscopic skull base surgery (ESBS) in real-time to assist in visualizing blood vessels and tumors [92]. These agents work by exciting electrons by absorbing high-energy light and emitting lower-energy light as the electrons return to their ground state. Fluorescence agents can differentiate tumors from healthy tissue, aiding in more precise tumor resection [93]. One commonly used fluorescence agent is indocyanine green (ICG), which binds to plasma proteins in the blood vessels and has a favorable safety profile [94]. It is used to visualize and avoid damage to blood vessels during surgery. ICG has also been studied in various tumors, including pituitary adenoma. Fluorescence intensity measured shortly after ICG infusion can distinguish healthy tissue from a pituitary adenoma. Another technique involves the infusion of high-dose ICG 24 hours before surgery, known as second-window ICG, which concentrates fluorescence within the pituitary adenoma [95]. Another fluorescence agent, 5-aminolevulinic acid (5-ALA), is approved for intraoperative visualization of high-grade glioma. It acts through the porphyrin synthesis pathway and has been studied in ESBS for different conditions, although its utility appears to be limited in specific tumor types [96]. 5-ALA can improve the detection of tumor tissue near the optic canal, as the proximity of an endoscope to the tissue enhances fluorescent signal detection for deeply located pathologies. Further understanding of the properties and pharmacokinetics of 5-ALA specific to each lesion can enhance its use in ESBS [97]. On Target Laboratories (OTL)-38 is a fluorophore that targets folate receptor alpha. It shows promise in detecting tumors that overexpress folate receptors. In a prospective study, OTL-38 demonstrated high sensitivity and specificity in detecting nonfunctioning pituitary adenomas during surgery [98]. OTL-38 also improved the resection of tumor margins compared to visual inspection alone. However, a limitation of OTL-38 is the lack of preoperative knowledge about folate receptor expression levels, which may reduce sensitivity and increase false negative results [99]. Ongoing research focuses on these agents and other fluorophores, such as sodium fluorescein, to enhance visualization and improve patient outcomes in ESBS.

Although not widely adopted in ESBS, ultrasonography has been assessed for pituitary tumor resection, with limitations in evaluating complex skull base anatomy [100]. Smaller-sized probes with improved resolution have been developed, which may increase the utility of ultrasonography in ESBS. A retrospective study reported an improved extent of resection and fewer complications in patients who underwent ultrasound-guided pituitary adenoma resection compared to traditional surgery [101]. Color Doppler ultrasonography, which uses color to label fluid velocity, can identify vascular structures in the skull base, including the internal carotid artery. Recent advancements in probe portability and resolution have led to the development of color Doppler microvascular probes. These probes have shown promise in identifying critical vascular structures during ESBS [102]. However, image resolution and accurate structure identification still need to be improved. The use of ultrasound contrast agents may further enhance ultrasonography in ESBS.

Intraoperative CT and MRI have proven beneficial in assessing residual tumor tissue, leading to improved extent of resection and progression-free survival. These imaging techniques have been employed during surgery to evaluate skull base anatomy. Intraoperative CT can be performed using mobile units [103], while intraoperative MRI requires dedicated imaging suites. One advantage of intraoperative imaging is the ability to perform re-registration of the neuronavigation system during surgery, particularly useful in open cranial procedures where brain shift can occur. Re-registration provides real-time updated imaging information to the surgeon and helps identify changes in anatomical structures. However, there are limitations to intraoperative imaging in endoscopic skull base surgery [104]. MRI is time-consuming and can prolong surgery duration [105]. CT involves exposure to ionizing radiation, which limits its use in specific patient populations like children and pregnant women [106].

The exoscope has been developed as a telescopic intraoperative visualization device with high-definition (H.D.) video resolution [107 - 110]. Unlike the endoscope, the exoscope is positioned outside the patient's body. It provides greater magnification, a wider focal distance, image enhancement, and 3D visualization. These features improve anatomical visualization, enhance surgeon comfort and ergonomics, and facilitate teaching. Exoscopy is a relatively new advancement in skull base surgery, and further research is needed to understand its strengths and limitations [107, 109]. Some limitations include tissue differentiation, loss of stereoscopy, and the need for better integration with existing technologies like fluorescence agents and endoscopy. Combining endoscopes with exoscopes has shown improved visualization of blind spots during surgery. The exo-endoscopic approach offers a broader field of view [109], improved instrument positioning, and enhanced viewing perspective for shared observation by operating room personnel. Continued experience with the exo-endoscopic approach can advance the complementary use of these technologies in endoscopic skull base surgery.

Other forms of endoscope-assisted bimanual microsurgical techniques are emerging. As endoscopic instruments evolve and surgical techniques advance, the portfolio of endoscopy applications in neurosurgery will extend beyond intraventricular and skull base lesions to encompass intraparenchymal brain lesions as well. These advancements will play a crucial role in the future of endoscope-assisted microsurgery. More far fledged applications could include remote controlled robotic neurosurgery applications. Nanotechnology has found numerous applications in medicine and it is conceivable that it might aid in neuroendoscopy as well by changing the indications for minimal and ultraminimal access neurosurgery. The authors of this chapter expect that neuroendoscopy will become a routine practice in modern neurosurgical procedures in the coming years. Therefore, institutions should establish comprehensive training programs to prepare graduating neurosurgeons for this rapidly evolving field.

DISCUSSION

The evolution of neuroendoscopy owes much to technological advancements, facilitating advanced and more complex interventions within the cerebral and neuroaxial confines. Historically, the direct visualization and illumination techniques encompasses surgical loupes, headlights, microscopes, endoscopes, and exoscopes, each enabling neurosurgeons to move away from expansive craniotomies to refined keyhole and endonasal methodologies leveraging the innate nasal corridor to access the cranial base [81].

In contrast to conventional microscopic modalities, neuroendoscopy boasts superiorities such as amplified magnification, enhanced structural discernment, comprehensive views via angled optics, and adept navigation around pivotal neurovascular constructs, like the internal carotid arteries and cranial nerves [111]. Clinical evidence underscores its merits in terms of enhanced neurological function, epitomized in scenarios like visual field amplification in pituitary macroadenomas or optimal hypothalamic conservation in craniopharyngiomas. Postoperative metrics also indicate benefits such as abbreviated hospitalization and diminished patient distress vis-a-vis traditional microsurgical interventions [112]. Nevertheless, current neuroendoscopic approaches, confined by a bi-dimensional perspective, have optimal efficacy for more diminutive midline anomalies. When considering endoscopic skull base surgery (ESBS), one must note potential sequelae, such as cerebrospinal fluid rhinorrhea (8.9% incidence), vascular disruption, endocrine dysregulation (2.0%), neurosystemic infections (1.7%), and albeit infrequent, mortality (0.4%) [113]. Hence, ESBS warrants discerning deployment by adept cranial base specialists, tailored to individual patient pathologies.

Technological leaps in intraoperative imaging, notably with CT and MRI, proffer richer data while counteracting brain displacement for neuronavigation apparatuses. Enhanced registration precision during surgical procedures can elevate neuronavigational exactitude. Augmented reality-driven neuronavigation emerges as a potent tool for rendering precise, patient-centric anatomical elucidation, with real-time augmentations being invaluable for safeguarding eloquent cerebral zones. Advances in image computation and data archiving can curtail the computational overhead of digitized methodologies, serving dual purposes: offering novice practitioners simulation-based learning and supplementary anatomical insight. Wider access to cadaveric dissections, facilitated by dedicated labs and scholarly atlases, promises to broaden the shared understanding of cranial base anatomy.

CONCLUSIONS:

In summation, the technological basis of neuroendoscopy and specifically, skull base surgery, has witnessed monumental evolution, most notably with the advent of ultra-high-definition imaging and three-dimensional optics. Endoscopic applications have burgeoned, transcending traditional transnasal paradigms. The potential of fluorescence agents in discerning residual neoplastic tissues awaits validation. Innovations like contrast-enhanced ultrasonography necessitate rigorous evaluation for their prowess in pinpointing critical vasculature. Neuronavigation platforms furnish surgeons with precise anatomical blueprints for surgical strategizing and implementation. Virtual and augmented realities are reshaping surgical training, enhancing acquisition of surgical skills. Exoscopes emerge as supplementary tools for intraoperative inspection. The incipient stage of robotic interventions primarily hinges on equipment dimensions and the confined nature of the existing neuroendoscopic access portal to the cranial base. It behooves surgeons to be familiar with the capabilities and constraints of each visualization modality to maximize patient outcomes.

REFERENCES

[1]   Li KW, Nelson C, Suk I, Jallo GI. Neuroendoscopy: past, present, and future. Neurosurg Focus 2005; 19(6): 1-5.
       [http://dx.doi.org/10.3171/foc.2005.19.6.2] [PMID: 16398474]

[2]   Hsu W, Li KW, Bookland M, Jallo GI. Keyhole to the brain: Walter Dandy and neuroendoscopy. J Neurosurg Pediatr 2009; 3(5): 439-42.
       [http://dx.doi.org/10.3171/2009.1.PEDS08342] [PMID: 19409026]

[3]   Mixter WJ. Ventriculoscopy and puncture of the floor of the third ventricle: Preliminary report of a case. Boston Med Surg J 1923; 188(9): 277-8.
       [http://dx.doi.org/10.1056/NEJM192303011880909]

[4]   Walker ML. History of Ventriculostomy. Neurosurg Clin N Am 2001; 12(1): 101-110, viii.
       [http://dx.doi.org/10.1016/S1042-3680(18)30070-6] [PMID: 11175991]

[5]   Nulsen FE, Spitz EB. Treatment of hydrocephalus by direct shunt from ventricle to jugular vain. Surg Forum 1951; •••: 399-403.
       [PMID: 14931257]

[6]   Vries JK. An endoscopic technique for third ventriculostomy. Surg Neurol 1978; 9(3): 165-8.
       [PMID: 635761]

[7]   Jones RF, Stening WA, Brydon M. Endoscopic third ventriculostomy. Neurosurgery. 1990; 26(1): 86-91; discussion-2.

[8]   Jones RFC, Kwok BCT, Stening WA, Vonau M. Neuroendoscopic third ventriculostomy. A practical alternative to extracranial shunts in non-communicating hydrocephalus. Acta Neurochir Suppl (Wien) 1994; 61: 79-83.
       [http://dx.doi.org/10.1007/978-3-7091-6908-7_14] [PMID: 7771230]

[9]   Jankowski R, Auque J, Simon C, Marchal JC, Hepner H, Wayoff M. How i do it: Head and neck and plastic surgery: Endoscopic pituitary tumor surgery. Laryngoscope 1992; 102(2): 198-202.
       [http://dx.doi.org/10.1288/00005537-199202000-00016] [PMID: 1738293]

[10]   Jho HD, Carrau RL. Endoscopic endonasal transsphenoidal surgery: experience with 50 patients. J Neurosurg 1997; 87(1): 44-51.
       [http://dx.doi.org/10.3171/jns.1997.87.1.0044] [PMID: 9202264]

[11]   Hopf NJ, Grunert P, Fries G, Resch KD, Perneczky A. Endoscopic third ventriculostomy: outcome analysis of 100 consecutive procedures. Neurosurgery. 1999; 44(4): 795-804; discussion-6.

[12]   Wellons JC III, Tubbs RS, Banks JT, *et al.* Long-term control of hydrocephalus via endoscopic third ventriculostomy in children with tectal plate gliomas. Neurosurgery 2002; 51(1): 63-8.
       [http://dx.doi.org/10.1097/00006123-200207000-00010] [PMID: 12182436]

[13]   Oi S, Abbott R. Loculated ventricles and isolated compartments in hydrocephalus: their pathophysiology and the efficacy of neuroendoscopic surgery. Neurosurg Clin N Am 2004; 15(1): 77-87.
       [http://dx.doi.org/10.1016/S1042-3680(03)00072-X] [PMID: 15062406]

[14]   Sgouros S. Neuroendoscopy: current status and future trends 2013.

[15]   Di Rocco F, Yoshino M, Oi S. Neuroendoscopic transventricular ventriculocystostomy in treatment for intracranial cysts. J Neurosurg 2005; 103(1) (Suppl.): 54-60.
[PMID: 16122006]

[16]   Fukushima T, Ishijima B, Hirakawa K, Nakamura N, Sano K. Ventriculofiberscope: a new technique for endoscopic diagnosis and operation. J Neurosurg 1973; 38(2): 251-6.
[http://dx.doi.org/10.3171/jns.1973.38.2.0251] [PMID: 4694225]

[17]   Yamini B, Refai D, Rubin CM, Frim DM. Initial endoscopic management of pineal region tumors and associated hydrocephalus: clinical series and literature review. J Neurosurg. 2004; 100(5 Suppl Pediatrics): 437-41.

[18]   Jimenez DF, Barone CM. Endoscopic craniectomy for early surgical correction of sagittal craniosynostosis. J Neurosurg 1998; 88(1): 77-81.
[http://dx.doi.org/10.3171/jns.1998.88.1.0077] [PMID: 9420076]

[19]   Jimenez DF, Barone CM, McGee ME, Cartwright CC, Baker CL. Endoscopy-assisted wide-vertex craniectomy, barrel stave osteotomies, and postoperative helmet molding therapy in the management of sagittal suture craniosynostosis. J Neurosurg. 2004; 100(5 Suppl Pediatrics): 407-17.

[20]   Rekate HL, Feiz-Erfan I, Ng YT, Gonzalez LF, Kerrigan JF. Endoscopic surgery for hypothalamic hamartomas causing medically refractory gelastic epilepsy. Childs Nerv Syst 2006; 22(8): 874-80.
[http://dx.doi.org/10.1007/s00381-006-0125-4] [PMID: 16770620]

[21]   Ishii K, Matsumoto M, Watanabe K, Nakamura M, Chiba K, Toyama Y. Endoscopic resection of cystic lesions in the lumbar spinal canal: a report of two cases. Minim Invasive Neurosurg 2005; 48(4): 240-3.
[http://dx.doi.org/10.1055/s-2005-870927] [PMID: 16172971]

[22]   Nagy I, Nádasi G, Széll K, Márkus B. Thoracic and lumbar sympathectomy with the application of ROMICRO mini laparotomy set. Acta Chir Hung 1997; 36(1-4): 246-7.
[PMID: 9408361]

[23]   Liu W, Li Q, Li Z, Chen L, Tian D, Jing J. Clinical efficacy of percutaneous transforaminal endoscopic discectomy in treating adolescent lumbar disc herniation. Medicine (Baltimore) 2019; 98(9): e14682.
[http://dx.doi.org/10.1097/MD.0000000000014682] [PMID: 30817599]

[24]   Lewandrowski KU, Ransom NA. Five-year clinical outcomes with endoscopic transforaminal outside-in foraminoplasty techniques for symptomatic degenerative conditions of the lumbar spine. J Spine Surg 2020; 6(S1) (Suppl. 1): S54-65.
[http://dx.doi.org/10.21037/jss.2019.07.03] [PMID: 32195416]

[25]   Pan M, Li Q, Li S, *et al.* Percutaneous Endoscopic Lumbar Discectomy: Indications and Complications. Pain Physician 2020; 23(1): 49-56.
[PMID: 32013278]

[26]   Ramírez León JF, Rugeles Ortíz JG, Martínez CR, Alonso Cuéllar GO, Lewandrowski KU. Surgical treatment of cervical radiculopathy using an anterior cervical endoscopic decompression. J Spine Surg 2020; 6(S1) (Suppl. 1): S179-85.
[http://dx.doi.org/10.21037/jss.2019.09.24] [PMID: 32195426]

[27]   Yeung A, Lewandrowski KU. Five-year clinical outcomes with endoscopic transforaminal foraminoplasty for symptomatic degenerative conditions of the lumbar spine: a comparative study of *inside-out* versus *outside-in* techniques. J Spine Surg 2020; 6(S1) (Suppl. 1): S66-83.
[http://dx.doi.org/10.21037/jss.2019.06.08] [PMID: 32195417]

[28]   Zou H, Hu Y, Liu J, Wu J. Percutaneous Endoscopic Transforaminal Lumbar Discectomy *via* Eccentric Trepan foraminoplasty Technology for Unilateral Stenosed Serve Root Canals. Orthop Surg 2020; 12(4): 1205-11.
[http://dx.doi.org/10.1111/os.12739] [PMID: 32857925]

[29]   Khoo LT, Palmer S, Laich DT, Fessler RG. Minimally invasive percutaneous posterior lumbar interbody fusion. Neurosurgery 2002; 51(5) (Suppl. 2): S2-166-, S2-181.
[http://dx.doi.org/10.1097/00006123-200211002-00023] [PMID: 12234445]

[30]   Ahn Y, Keum HJ, Shin SH. Percutaneous Endoscopic Cervical Discectomy versus Anterior Cervical Discectomy and Fusion: A Comparative Cohort Study with a Five-Year Follow-Up. J Clin Med 2020; 9(2): 371.
[http://dx.doi.org/10.3390/jcm9020371] [PMID: 32013206]

[31]   Tacconi L, Giordan E. A Novel Hybrid Endoscopic Approach for Anterior Cervical Discectomy and Fusion and a Meta-Analysis of the Literature. World Neurosurg 2019; 131: e237-46.
[http://dx.doi.org/10.1016/j.wneu.2019.07.122] [PMID: 31349080]

[32]   Du Q, Lei LQ, Cao GR, *et al.* Percutaneous full-endoscopic anterior transcorporeal cervical discectomy and channel repair: a technique note report. BMC Musculoskelet Disord 2019; 20(1): 280.
[http://dx.doi.org/10.1186/s12891-019-2659-0] [PMID: 31182078]

[33]   Heo DH, Son SK, Eum JH, Park CK. Fully endoscopic lumbar interbody fusion using a percutaneous unilateral biportal endoscopic technique: technical note and preliminary clinical results. Neurosurg Focus 2017; 43(2): E8.
[http://dx.doi.org/10.3171/2017.5.FOCUS17146] [PMID: 28760038]

[34]   Fonoff ET, Lopez WOC, de Oliveira YSA, Lara NA, Teixeira MJ. Endoscopic approaches to the spinal cord. Acta Neurochir Suppl (Wien) 2011; 108: 75-84.
[http://dx.doi.org/10.1007/978-3-211-99370-5_12] [PMID: 21107941]

[35]   Bergamaschi JPM, Costa CAM, Sandon LH. Full-Endoscopic Resection of Osteoid Osteoma in the Thoracic Spine: A Case Report. Int J Spine Surg 2021; 14(s4): S78-86.
[http://dx.doi.org/10.14444/7169] [PMID: 33900949]

[36]   Hagan MJ, Telfeian AE, Sastry R, *et al.* Awake transforaminal endoscopic lumbar facet cyst resection: technical note and case series. J Neurosurg Spine 2022; 37(6): 843-50.
[http://dx.doi.org/10.3171/2022.6.SPINE22451] [PMID: 35986734]

[37]   Alkhaibary A, Baydhi L, Alharbi A, *et al.* Endoscopic versus Open Microsurgical Excision of Colloid Cysts: A Comparative Analysis and State-of-the-Art Review of Neurosurgical Techniques. World Neurosurg 2021; 149: e298-308.
[http://dx.doi.org/10.1016/j.wneu.2021.02.032] [PMID: 33601083]

[38]   Sharma SB, Lin GX, Jabri H, Siddappa ND, Kim JS. Biportal Endoscopic Excision of Facetal Cyst in the Far Lateral Region of L5S1: 2-Dimensional Operative Video. Oper Neurosurg (Hagerstown) 2020; 18(6): E233.
[http://dx.doi.org/10.1093/ons/opz255] [PMID: 31504842]

[39]   Yeung AT, Yeung CA. In-vivo endoscopic visualization of patho-anatomy in painful degenerative conditions of the lumbar spine. Surg Technol Int 2006; 15: 243-56.
[PMID: 17029183]

[40]   An B, Li XC, Zhou CP, *et al.* Percutaneous full endoscopic posterior decompression of thoracic myelopathy caused by ossification of the ligamentum flavum. Eur Spine J 2019; 28(3): 492-501.
[http://dx.doi.org/10.1007/s00586-018-05866-2] [PMID: 30656471]

[41]   Ruetten S, Hahn P, Oezdemir S, *et al.* Full-endoscopic uniportal decompression in disc herniations and stenosis of the thoracic spine using the interlaminar, extraforaminal, or transthoracic retropleural approach. J Neurosurg Spine 2018; 29(2): 157-68.
[http://dx.doi.org/10.3171/2017.12.SPINE171096] [PMID: 29856303]

[42]   Ruetten S, Hahn P, Oezdemir S, Baraliakos X, Godolias G, Komp M. Operation of Soft or Calcified Thoracic Disc Herniations in the Full-Endoscopic Uniportal Extraforaminal Technique. Pain Physician 2018; 1(21;1): E331-40.
[http://dx.doi.org/10.36076/ppj.2018.4.E331] [PMID: 30045599]

[43]   Ruetten S, Hahn P, Oezdemir S, Baraliakos X, Godolias G, Komp M. Decompression of the anterior thoracic spinal canal using a novel full□endoscopic uniportal transthoracic retropleural technique—an anatomical feasibility study in human cadavers. Clin Anat 2018; 31(5): 716-23.
[http://dx.doi.org/10.1002/ca.23075] [PMID: 29577428]

[44]   Haufe SMW, Baker RA, Pyne ML. Endoscopic thoracic laminoforaminoplasty for the treatment of thoracic radiculopathy: report of 12 cases. Int J Med Sci 2009; 6(4): 224-6.
[http://dx.doi.org/10.7150/ijms.6.224] [PMID: 19742241]

[45]   Lewandrowski KU, Telfeian AE, Hellinger S, *et al*. Difficulties, Challenges, and the Learning Curve of Avoiding Complications in Lumbar Endoscopic Spine Surgery. Int J Spine Surg 2021; 15 (Suppl. 3): S21-37.
[http://dx.doi.org/10.14444/8161] [PMID: 34974418]

[46]   Kim JE, Yoo HS, Choi DJ, Park EJ, Jee SM. Comparison of Minimal Invasive Versus Biportal Endoscopic Transforaminal Lumbar Interbody Fusion for Single-level Lumbar Disease. Clin Spine Surg 2021; 34(2): E64-71.
[http://dx.doi.org/10.1097/BSD.0000000000001024] [PMID: 33633061]

[47]   Ito Z, Shibayama M, Nakamura S, *et al*. Clinical Comparison of Unilateral Biportal Endoscopic Laminectomy versus Microendoscopic Laminectomy for Single-Level Laminectomy: A Single-Center, Retrospective Analysis. World Neurosurg 2021; 148: e581-8.
[http://dx.doi.org/10.1016/j.wneu.2021.01.031] [PMID: 33476779]

[48]   Gadjradj PS, Harhangi BS, Amelink J, *et al*. Percutaneous Transforaminal Endoscopic Discectomy Versus Open Microdiscectomy for Lumbar Disc Herniation. Spine 2021; 46(8): 538-49.
[http://dx.doi.org/10.1097/BRS.0000000000003843] [PMID: 33290374]

[49]   Avellanal M, Diaz-Reganon G, Orts A, Gonzalez-Montero L, Riquelme I. Transforaminal Epiduroscopy in Patients with Failed Back Surgery Syndrome. Pain Physician 2019; 1(22;1): 89-95.
[http://dx.doi.org/10.36076/ppj/2019.22.89] [PMID: 30700072]

[50]   Hazer DB, Acarbaş A, Rosberg HE. The outcome of epiduroscopy treatment in patients with chronic low back pain and radicular pain, operated or non-operated for lumbar disc herniation: a retrospective study in 88 patients. Korean J Pain 2018; 31(2): 109-15.
[http://dx.doi.org/10.3344/kjp.2018.31.2.109] [PMID: 29686809]

[51]   Avellanal M, Diaz-Reganon G. Interlaminar approach for epiduroscopy in patients with failed back surgery syndrome. Br J Anaesth 2008; 101(2): 244-9.
[http://dx.doi.org/10.1093/bja/aen165] [PMID: 18552347]

[52]   Ruetten S, Meyer O, Godolias G. Endoscopic surgery of the lumbar epidural space (epiduroscopy): results of therapeutic intervention in 93 patients. Minim Invasive Neurosurg 2003; 46(1): 1-4.
[http://dx.doi.org/10.1055/s-2003-37962] [PMID: 12640575]

[53]   Conger AR, Lucas J, Zada G, Schwartz TH, Cohen-Gadol AA. Endoscopic extended transsphenoidal resection of craniopharyngiomas: nuances of neurosurgical technique. Neurosurg Focus 2014; 37(4): E10.
[http://dx.doi.org/10.3171/2014.7.FOCUS14364] [PMID: 25270129]

[54]   Steineke TC, Barbery D. Extended reality platform for minimally invasive endoscopic evacuation of deep-seated intracerebral hemorrhage: illustrative case. Journal of Neurosurgery: Case Lessons 2022; 4(12): CASE21390.
[http://dx.doi.org/10.3171/CASE21390] [PMID: 36593677]

[55]   Carrau RL, Jho HD, Ko Y. Transnasal-transsphenoidal endoscopic surgery of the pituitary gland. Laryngoscope 1996; 106(7): 914-8.
[http://dx.doi.org/10.1097/00005537-199607000-00025] [PMID: 8667994]

[56]   Cappabianca P, Alfieri A, Stefano T, Buonamassa S, Enrico D. Instruments for endoscopic endonasal transsphenoidal surgery. Neurosurgery 1999; 45(2): 392-5.

[http://dx.doi.org/10.1097/00006123-199908000-00041] [PMID: 10449087]

[57]   Batra PS, Lee J, Barnett SL, Senior BA, Setzen M, Kraus DH. Endoscopic skull base surgery practice patterns: survey of the North American Skull Base Society. Int Forum Allergy Rhinol 2013; 3(8): 659-63.
[http://dx.doi.org/10.1002/alr.21151] [PMID: 23389885]

[58]   Martinez-Perez R, Hardesty DA, Silveira-Bertazzo G, Albonette-Felicio T, Carrau RL, Prevedello DM. Safety and effectiveness of endoscopic endonasal intracranial aneurysm clipping: a systematic review. Neurosurg Rev 2021; 44(2): 889-96.
[http://dx.doi.org/10.1007/s10143-020-01316-0] [PMID: 32458275]

[59]   Battaglia P, Lambertoni A, Castelnuovo P. Transnasal Endoscopic Surgery: Surgical Techniques and Complications. Adv Otorhinolaryngol 2020; 84: 46-55.
[http://dx.doi.org/10.1159/000457924] [PMID: 32731234]

[60]   Buchlak QD, Esmaili N, Bennett C, Wang YY, King J, Goldschlager T. Predictors of improvement in quality of life at 12-month follow-up in patients undergoing anterior endoscopic skull base surgery. PLoS One 2022; 17(7): e0272147.
[http://dx.doi.org/10.1371/journal.pone.0272147] [PMID: 35895728]

[61]   Butenschoen VM, Wostrack M, Meyer B, Gempt J. Endoscopic Transnasal Odontoidectomy for Ventral Decompression of the Craniovertebral Junction: Surgical Technique and Clinical Outcome in a Case Series of 19 Patients. Oper Neurosurg (Hagerstown) 2021; 20(1): 24-31.
[http://dx.doi.org/10.1093/ons/opaa331] [PMID: 33094804]

[62]   Conrad J, Blaese M, Becker S, Huppertz T, Ayyad A, Ringel F. Sinonasal Outcome After Endoscopic Transnasal Surgery—A Prospective Rhinological Study. Oper Neurosurg (Hagerstown) 2023; 24(3): 223-31.
[http://dx.doi.org/10.1227/ons.0000000000000532] [PMID: 36701557]

[63]   Ergen A, Caklili M, Uzuner A, *et al.* Endoscopically operated 15 ventral skull-base dermoid and epidermoid cysts: Outcomes of a case series and technical note. Neurochirurgie 2023; 69(2): 101424.
[http://dx.doi.org/10.1016/j.neuchi.2023.101424] [PMID: 36868134]

[64]   Gstrein NA, Zwicky S, Serra C, *et al.* Rhinologic outcome of endoscopic transnasal-transsphenoidal pituitary surgery: an institutional series, systematic review, and meta-analysis. Eur Arch Otorhinolaryngol 2023; 280(9): 4091-9.
[http://dx.doi.org/10.1007/s00405-023-07934-w] [PMID: 36988686]

[65]   Deopujari CE, Gupta PP, Shaikh ST, Shah N. Transnasal Endoscopic Surgery for Suprasellar Meningiomas. Neurol India 2021; 69(3): 630-5.
[http://dx.doi.org/10.4103/0028-3886.319224] [PMID: 34169857]

[66]   Kahilogullari G, Meco C, Beton S, *et al.* Endoscopic Transnasal Skull Base Surgery in Pediatric Patients. J Neurol Surg B Skull Base 2020; 81(5): 515-25.
[http://dx.doi.org/10.1055/s-0039-1692641] [PMID: 33134019]

[67]   Li H, Zhai X, He J, Zhang J, Liu G. [Surgical approach of transnasal endoscopic resection of benign lesions in the paramedian lateral skull base]. Lin Chuang Er Bi Yan Hou Tou Jing Wai Ke Za Zhi 2022; 36(5): 352-6. [Surgical approach of transnasal endoscopic resection of benign lesions in the paramedian lateral skull base].
[PMID: 35483685]

[68]   Li L, London NR Jr, Prevedello DM, Carrau RL. Endoscopic Endonasal Approach to the Pterygopalatine Fossa and Infratemporal Fossa: Comparison of the Prelacrimal and Denker's Corridors. Am J Rhinol Allergy 2022; 36(5): 599-606.
[http://dx.doi.org/10.1177/19458924221097159] [PMID: 35506931]

[69]   Liu J, Sun X, Liu Q, *et al.* A minimally invasive endoscopic transnasal retropterygoid approach to the upper parapharyngeal space: anatomic studies and surgical implications. Int Forum Allergy Rhinol 2019; 9(11): 1263-72.

[http://dx.doi.org/10.1002/alr.22437] [PMID: 31574593]

[70]   Martinez-Perez R, Aref M, Ramakhrisnan V, Youssef AS. Combined biportal unilateral endoscopic endonasal and endoscopic anterior transmaxillary approach for resection of lesions involving the infratemporal fossa. Acta Neurochir (Wien) 2021; 163(12): 3439-45.
[http://dx.doi.org/10.1007/s00701-021-04994-x] [PMID: 34633545]

[71]   Silveira-Bertazzo G, Manjila S, Carrau RL, Prevedello DM. Expanded endoscopic endonasal approach for extending suprasellar and third ventricular lesions. Acta Neurochir (Wien) 2020; 162(10): 2403-8.
[http://dx.doi.org/10.1007/s00701-020-04368-9] [PMID: 32385641]

[72]   Singh R, Thorwarth R, Bendok BR, Lal D. Endoscopic Endonasal and Transmaxillary Resection of a Nasopharyngeal Angiofibroma. World Neurosurg 2021; 155: 180.
[http://dx.doi.org/10.1016/j.wneu.2021.08.064] [PMID: 34450322]

[73]   Todeschini AB, Beer-Furlan A, Otto B, Prevedello DM, Carrau RL. Endoscopic Endonasal Approaches for Anterior Skull Base Meningiomas. Adv Otorhinolaryngol 2020; 84: 114-23.
[http://dx.doi.org/10.1159/000457931] [PMID: 32731224]

[74]   Vedhapoodi A, Periyasamy A, Senthilkumar D. A novel combined transorbital transnasal endoscopic approach for reconstruction of posttraumatic complex anterior cranial fossa defect. Asian J Neurosurg 2021; 16(1): 136-40.
[http://dx.doi.org/10.4103/ajns.AJNS_363_20] [PMID: 34211881]

[75]   Wang Y, Jin C, Cui N, Yang J. Transnasal Endoscopy and Combined Approach to Infratemporal Fossa Abscess and Parapharyngeal Abscess. J Craniofac Surg 2022; 33(8): 2534-7.
[http://dx.doi.org/10.1097/SCS.0000000000008798] [PMID: 35905380]

[76]   Xin G, Liu Y, Xiong Y, *et al.* The use of three-dimensional endoscope in transnasal skull base surgery: A single-center experience from China. Front Surg 2022; 9: 996290.
[http://dx.doi.org/10.3389/fsurg.2022.996290] [PMID: 36211263]

[77]   Zhang C, Yang Z, Liu P. Strategy of skull base reconstruction after endoscopic transnasal pituitary adenoma resection. Front Surg 2023; 10: 1130660.
[http://dx.doi.org/10.3389/fsurg.2023.1130660] [PMID: 36998598]

[78]   Zhang H, Gao KL, Xie ZH, *et al.* [Clinical study on endoscopic surgery for soft tissue necrosis of cranial base after radiotherapy for nasopharyngeal carcinoma]. Zhonghua Er Bi Yan Hou Tou Jing Wai Ke Za Zhi 2021; 56(1): 26-32. [Clinical study on endoscopic surgery for soft tissue necrosis of cranial base after radiotherapy for nasopharyngeal carcinoma].
[PMID: 33472299]

[79]   Boese A, Wex C, Croner R, *et al.* Endoscopic Imaging Technology Today. Diagnostics (Basel) 2022; 12(5): 1262.
[http://dx.doi.org/10.3390/diagnostics12051262] [PMID: 35626417]

[80]   Jarmula J, de Andrade EJ, Kshettry VR, Recinos PF. The Current State of Visualization Techniques in Endoscopic Skull Base Surgery. Brain Sci 2022; 12(10): 1337.
[http://dx.doi.org/10.3390/brainsci12101337] [PMID: 36291271]

[81]   Riley CA, Soneru CP, Tabaee A, Kacker A, Anand VK, Schwartz TH. Technological and Ideological Innovations in Endoscopic Skull Base Surgery. World Neurosurg 2019; 124: 513-21.
[http://dx.doi.org/10.1016/j.wneu.2019.01.120] [PMID: 30708082]

[82]   Balogun JA, Daniel A, Idowu OK. Navigating the learning curve with large and giant tumors: Initial experience with endoscopic endonasal transphenoidal resection of PitNETs. J Clin Neurosci 2023; 112: 6-11.
[http://dx.doi.org/10.1016/j.jocn.2023.04.001] [PMID: 37023497]

[83]   Boaro A, Moscolo F, Feletti A, *et al.* Visualization, navigation, augmentation. The ever-changing perspective of the neurosurgeon. Brain and Spine 2022; 2: 100926.
[http://dx.doi.org/10.1016/j.bas.2022.100926] [PMID: 36248169]

[84] Thomas NWD, Sinclair J. Image-Guided Neurosurgery: History and Current Clinical Applications. J Med Imaging Radiat Sci 2015; 46(3): 331-42.
[http://dx.doi.org/10.1016/j.jmir.2015.06.003] [PMID: 31052141]

[85] Mishra R, Narayanan MDK, Umana GE, Montemurro N, Chaurasia B, Deora H. Virtual Reality in Neurosurgery: Beyond Neurosurgical Planning. Int J Environ Res Public Health 2022; 19(3): 1719.
[http://dx.doi.org/10.3390/ijerph19031719] [PMID: 35162742]

[86] Zeiger J, Costa A, Bederson J, Shrivastava RK, Iloreta AMC. Use of Mixed Reality Visualization in Endoscopic Endonasal Skull Base Surgery. Oper Neurosurg (Hagerstown) 2020; 19(1): 43-52.
[http://dx.doi.org/10.1093/ons/opz355] [PMID: 31807786]

[87] Carl B, Bopp M, Voellger B, Saß B, Nimsky C. Augmented Reality in Transsphenoidal Surgery. World Neurosurg 2019; 125: e873-83.
[http://dx.doi.org/10.1016/j.wneu.2019.01.202] [PMID: 30763743]

[88] Lai M, Skyrman S, Shan C, *et al.* Fusion of augmented reality imaging with the endoscopic view for endonasal skull base surgery; a novel application for surgical navigation based on intraoperative cone beam computed tomography and optical tracking. PLoS One 2020; 15(1): e0227312.
[http://dx.doi.org/10.1371/journal.pone.0227312] [PMID: 31945082]

[89] Ashour R, Reintjes S, Park MS, Sivakanthan S, van Loveren H, Agazzi S. Intraoperative Magnetic Resonance Imaging in Skull Base Surgery: A Review of 71 Consecutive Cases. World Neurosurg 2016; 93: 183-90.
[http://dx.doi.org/10.1016/j.wneu.2016.06.045] [PMID: 27319315]

[90] James J, Irace AL, Gudis DA, Overdevest JB. Simulation training in endoscopic skull base surgery: A scoping review. World J Otorhinolaryngol Head Neck Surg 2022; 8(1): 73-81.
[http://dx.doi.org/10.1002/wjo2.11] [PMID: 35619934]

[91] Paro MR, Hersh DS, Bulsara KR. History of Virtual Reality and Augmented Reality in Neurosurgical Training. World Neurosurg 2022; 167: 37-43.
[http://dx.doi.org/10.1016/j.wneu.2022.08.042] [PMID: 35977681]

[92] Miner RC. Image-Guided Neurosurgery. J Med Imaging Radiat Sci 2017; 48(4): 328-35.
[http://dx.doi.org/10.1016/j.jmir.2017.06.005] [PMID: 31047466]

[93] Lakomkin N, Van Gompel JJ, Post KD, Cho SS, Lee JYK, Hadjipanayis CG. Fluorescence guided surgery for pituitary adenomas. J Neurooncol 2021; 151(3): 403-13.
[http://dx.doi.org/10.1007/s11060-020-03420-z] [PMID: 33611707]

[94] Reinhart MB, Huntington CR, Blair LJ, Heniford BT, Augenstein VA. Indocyanine Green. Surg Innov 2016; 23(2): 166-75.
[http://dx.doi.org/10.1177/1553350615604053] [PMID: 26359355]

[95] Jeon JW, Cho SS, Nag S, *et al.* Near-Infrared Optical Contrast of Skull Base Tumors During Endoscopic Endonasal Surgery. Oper Neurosurg (Hagerstown) 2019; 17(1): 32-42.
[http://dx.doi.org/10.1093/ons/opy213] [PMID: 30124919]

[96] Hadjipanayis CG, Stummer W. 5-ALA and FDA approval for glioma surgery. J Neurooncol 2019; 141(3): 479-86.
[http://dx.doi.org/10.1007/s11060-019-03098-y] [PMID: 30644008]

[97] Recinos PF. Editorial. Is the use of 5-ALA in endoscopic skull base surgery truly limited or in need of more refined evaluation? J Neurosurg 2021; 135(2): 532-3.
[http://dx.doi.org/10.3171/2020.7.JNS201870] [PMID: 33126207]

[98] Cho SS, Jeon J, Buch L, *et al.* Intraoperative near-infrared imaging with receptor-specific versus passive delivery of fluorescent agents in pituitary adenomas. J Neurosurg 2019; 131(6): 1974-84.
[http://dx.doi.org/10.3171/2018.7.JNS181642] [PMID: 30554181]

[99] Zhang DY, Singhal S, Lee JYK. Optical Principles of Fluorescence-Guided Brain Tumor Surgery: A

Practical Primer for the Neurosurgeon. Neurosurgery 2019; 85(3): 312-24.
[http://dx.doi.org/10.1093/neuros/nyy315] [PMID: 30085129]

[100] Machado I, Toews M, Luo J, *et al.* Non-rigid registration of 3D ultrasound for neurosurgery using automatic feature detection and matching. Int J CARS 2018; 13(10): 1525-38.
[http://dx.doi.org/10.1007/s11548-018-1786-7] [PMID: 29869321]

[101] Alshareef M, Lowe S, Park Y, Frankel B. Utility of intraoperative ultrasonography for resection of pituitary adenomas: a comparative retrospective study. Acta Neurochir (Wien) 2021; 163(6): 1725-34.
[http://dx.doi.org/10.1007/s00701-020-04674-2] [PMID: 33403430]

[102] AlQahtani A, Castelnuovo P, Nicolai P, Prevedello DM, Locatelli D, Carrau RL. Injury of the Internal Carotid Artery During Endoscopic Skull Base Surgery. Otolaryngol Clin North Am 2016; 49(1): 237-52.
[http://dx.doi.org/10.1016/j.otc.2015.09.009] [PMID: 26614841]

[103] Perin A, Carone G, Rui CB, *et al.* The "STARS–CT-MADE" Study: Advanced Rehearsal and Intraoperative Navigation for Skull Base Tumors. World Neurosurg 2021; 154: e19-28.
[http://dx.doi.org/10.1016/j.wneu.2021.06.058] [PMID: 34157459]

[104] Ueberschaer M, Vettermann FJ, Forbrig R, *et al.* Simpson Grade Revisited – Intraoperative Estimation of the Extent of Resection in Meningiomas Versus Postoperative Somatostatin Receptor Positron Emission Tomography/Computed Tomography and Magnetic Resonance Imaging. Neurosurgery 2021; 88(1): 140-6.
[http://dx.doi.org/10.1093/neuros/nyaa333] [PMID: 32827256]

[105] Sylvester PT, Evans JA, Zipfel GJ, *et al.* Combined high-field intraoperative magnetic resonance imaging and endoscopy increase extent of resection and progression-free survival for pituitary adenomas. Pituitary 2015; 18(1): 72-85.
[http://dx.doi.org/10.1007/s11102-014-0560-2] [PMID: 24599833]

[106] Tomà P, Bartoloni A, Salerno S, *et al.* Protecting sensitive patient groups from imaging using ionizing radiation: effects during pregnancy, in fetal life and childhood. Radiol Med (Torino) 2019; 124(8): 736-44.
[http://dx.doi.org/10.1007/s11547-019-01034-8] [PMID: 30949891]

[107] Acha JL, Contreras L, Lopez K, *et al.* Neurovascular Microsurgical Experience Through 3-Dimensional Exoscopy: Case Report and Literature Review. World Neurosurg 2023; 174: 63-8.
[http://dx.doi.org/10.1016/j.wneu.2023.02.120] [PMID: 36871654]

[108] Porto E, Revuelta-Barbero JM, Soriano RM, *et al.* Exoscope-Assisted Middle Cranial Fossa Approach for Repair of Tegmental Defects: A Cadaveric and Clinical Study. World Neurosurg 2022; 168: 103-10.
[http://dx.doi.org/10.1016/j.wneu.2022.09.096] [PMID: 36174947]

[109] Shibano A, Kimura H, Tatehara S, *et al.* Efficacy of a High-definition Three-dimensional Exoscope in Simultaneous Transcranial and Endoscopic Endonasal Surgery: A Case Report. NMC Case Rep J 2022; 9(0): 243-7.
[http://dx.doi.org/10.2176/jns-nmc.2022-0081] [PMID: 36128056]

[110] Zhang BY, Ho VWY, Tsai TY, Chan KC. An early report of exoscope-assisted otologic surgery. J Chin Med Assoc 2023; 86(5): 523-8.
[http://dx.doi.org/10.1097/JCMA.0000000000000907] [PMID: 36854146]

[111] Kasemsiri P, Carrau RL, Ditzel Filho LFS, *et al.* Advantages and limitations of endoscopic endonasal approaches to the skull base. World Neurosurg 2014; 82(6) (Suppl.): S12-21.
[http://dx.doi.org/10.1016/j.wneu.2014.07.022] [PMID: 25496622]

[112] Martinez-Perez R, Requena LC, Carrau RL, Prevedello DM. Modern endoscopic skull base neurosurgery. J Neurooncol 2021; 151(3): 461-75.
[http://dx.doi.org/10.1007/s11060-020-03610-9] [PMID: 33611712]

[113] Borg A, Kirkman MA, Choi D. Endoscopic Endonasal Anterior Skull Base Surgery: A Systematic Review of Complications During the Past 65 Years. World Neurosurg 2016; 95: 383-91.
[http://dx.doi.org/10.1016/j.wneu.2015.12.105] [PMID: 26960277]

CHAPTER 2

Trigeminal Tractotomies and Nucleotomies

William Omar Contreras López[1,*], Kai-Uwe Lewandrowski[2,3,4], Jorge Felipe Ramírez León[5,6,7] and Erich Talamoni Fonoff[8]

[1] *Clínica Foscal Internacional, Autopista Floridablanca - Girón, Km 7, Floridablanca, Santander, Colombia*

[2] *Center for Advanced Spine Care of Southern Arizona and Surgical Institute of Tucson, Tucson, AZ, USA*

[3] *Departmemt of Orthopaedics, Fundación Universitaria Sanitas, Bogotá, D.C., Colombia*

[4] *Department of Neurosurgery in the Video-Endoscopic Postgraduate Program at the Universidade Federal do Estado do Rio de Janeiro - UNIRIO, Rio de Janeiro, Brazil*

[5] *Minimally Invasive Spine Center. Bogotá, D.C., Colombia*

[6] *Reina Sofía Clinic. Bogotá, D.C., Colombia*

[7] *Fundación Universitaria Sanitas. Bogotá, D.C., Colombia*

[8] *Division of Functional Neurosurgery of Institute of Psychiatry, Department of Neurology, University of São Paulo Medical School, São Paulo, Brazil*

Abstract: Microendoscopic trigeminal nucleotractotomy (MENT) is a minimally invasive surgical procedure used to treat trigeminal neuralgia (TN). In this chapter, the authors describe the clinical outcomes associated with MENT regarding pain relief and functional improvement. Our novel technique resulted in a significant reduction in pain scores following MENT, as indicated by a decrease in the Visual Analog Scale (VAS) scores. Additionally, a substantial proportion of patients reported functional improvement, including enhanced ability to perform daily activities. The success of MENT is influenced by factors such as patient selection, surgical technique, and underlying causes of TN. Although the study provides short-term follow-up and feasibility data, further research with longer-term evaluations is necessary to assess the durability of pain relief achieved through MENT.

Keywords: Intractable pain, Microendoscopic, Trigeminal nucleotractotomy, Trigeminal neuralgia.

* **Corresponding author William Omar Contreras López:** Clínica Foscal Internacional, Autopista Floridablanca - Girón, Km 7, Floridablanca, Santander, Colombia; Tel: +573112957003; E-mail: wcontreras127@unab.edu.co

INTRODUCTION

Trigeminal tractotomies and nucleotomies are surgical procedures performed to alleviate severe and intractable pain associated with trigeminal neuralgia, a debilitating condition characterized by sudden, intense facial pain. These procedures aim to disrupt or remove the nerve fibers involved in transmitting pain signals along the trigeminal nerve pathway. While both tractotomy and nucleotomy target the trigeminal nerve, they differ in their approaches and techniques.

Trigeminal tractotomy is a surgical procedure that involves the selective lesioning or cutting of specific nerve tracts within the trigeminal nerve. The goal is to interrupt the transmission of pain signals from the affected area to the brain, thereby providing pain relief. Tractotomy procedures can be performed through several approaches, including percutaneous techniques using radiofrequency ablation, glycerol injections, or balloon compression. More invasive approaches, such as microvascular decompression or stereotactic radiosurgery, may also be utilized.

A related procedure, trigeminal nucleotomy, is a surgical intervention that involves the partial or complete removal of a section of the trigeminal nerve nucleus, which is the central part of the trigeminal nerve within the brainstem. This procedure aims to directly interrupt the pain signals at their source by removing or damaging the nerve cells responsible for transmitting pain sensations. Trigeminal nucleotomy is typically performed using microsurgical techniques and requires a high level of precision to avoid damaging adjacent structures and minimize potential complications.

Both trigeminal tractotomy and nucleotomy have demonstrated effectiveness in providing pain relief for patients with severe trigeminal neuralgia. However, these procedures are considered last-resort options when other more conservative treatments, such as medications or nerve blocks, have failed to adequately control the pain. They are generally reserved for patients with severe, refractory pain who have exhausted all other treatment options.

While trigeminal tractotomies and nucleotomies can provide significant pain relief, they are not without potential risks and complications. Common complications associated with these procedures include sensory loss, facial numbness, weakness, infection, and cerebrospinal fluid leaks. The decision to undertake these procedures requires a thorough evaluation of the patient's individual circumstances, including the severity of pain, overall health, and potential risks and benefits. The use of image-guided navigation systems, intraoperative monitoring, and refined surgical approaches has enhanced precision and reduced the risk of complications. Additionally, ongoing research aims to further optimize the selection criteria for these procedures and explore novel techniques, such as minimally invasive approaches and neurostimulation, to improve patient outcomes. In this chapter, the authors present the recent advances

in neurosurgical techniques and technologies, and their associated outcomes and safety profiles, with regard to trigeminal tractotomies and nucleotomies.

History

In 1937, Sjoqvist delineated an innovative approach wherein the trigeminal nerve's spinal tract could be meticulously sectioned *via* an incision on the posterolateral quadrant of the medulla, situated superiorly to the obex reference point [6]. Such an intervention typically culminated in ipsilateral thermoanalgesia confined to the facial region while preserving alternate sensation modalities [1]. Subsequent animal-based research and human surgical outcomes corroborated these preliminary findings. The technique gained traction, largely attributed to its reduced propensity to induce facial dysesthesias as compared to trigeminal rhizotomies [2]. Sjoqvist instituted this surgical strategy with the patient in a prone position, under the effect of general anesthesia. Following a suboccipital craniotomy, subsequent openings of the dura mater and arachnoid membrane were performed. The cerebellar tonsil was then gently retracted to afford optimal medullary visualization. The olive's anatomical prominence acted as the guiding landmark. Consequently, the trigeminal tract's incision was precisely executed a few millimeters posterior to the terminal vagal rootlet, to a depth range of 3.5–4 mm and situated 8–10 mm superior to the obex, in a domain enveloped by the restiform body (Fig. 1).

The procedure was challenging and led to numerous complications, including ipsilateral ataxia, damage to the recurrent laryngeal nerve, lateropulsion, contralateral analgesia, vocal cord paralysis, gait anomalies, and limb postural sensibility issues. The most significant complications of the trigeminal tractotomy arose from injuries to the restiform body and the nucleus ambiguus. Later, Grant unintentionally created a lesion beneath Sjoqvist's suggested level, resulting in analgesia across all three ipsilateral branches of the trigeminal nerve. This discovery led him to conclude that making lesions further from Sjoqvist's proposed area reduced complications. Thus, the lower part of the medulla and upper cervical cord emerged as the favored locations for trigeminal tractotomy, especially since cuts made at or below the obex could avoid damaging the spinocerebellar fibers.

Trigeminal tractotomy, while pioneering, was not devoid of complications. A notable proportion, over 60% of the initial patient cohort, exhibited ataxia, predominantly attributed to lesions within the spinocerebellar tract, particularly when the tract sectioning neared the obex [1]. Refinements in the original surgical methodology notably reduced the incidence of such ataxia to a minimal 5%. Occasionally, postoperative outcomes revealed an expanded scope of analgesia. Such manifestations saw thermoanalgesic regions spanning beyond the trigeminal boundary to territories governed by the upper cervical roots, inclusive of the seventh, ninth, and tenth cranial nerve domains. Vagal nerve lesions, identified in a range of 8-24% of the cohort, were particularly prevalent when the interventions were proximal to the obex. Interestingly, these lesions were less frequent when interventions targeted the trigeminal tract's distal segment. Horner's syndrome, cephalalgia, heightened anxiety, and emergent psychosis constituted the lesser prevalent complications. Mortality oscillated between 0 and 16.6%, with the lower threshold being observed in patients devoid of malignancies, and surging to an alarming 30% in those grappling with oncogenic pain etiologies [3, 5].

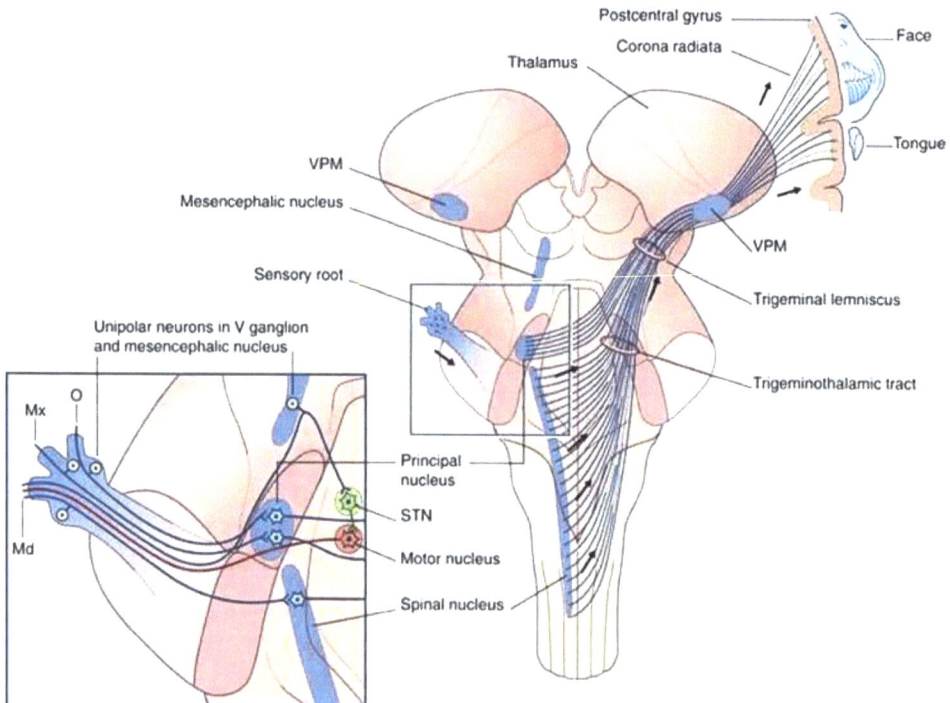

Fig. (1). The schematic diagram illustrates the anterolateral facets of the lower brain stem, highlighting the lesion location suggested by Sjoqvist and Grant. It delineates the association between the trigeminal tract, nucleus, and the restiform body in an open trigeminal tractotomy. An inset portrays the lower brain stem's posterior view, emphasizing the spatial relation between the trigeminal tract, nuclei, and the restiform body situated anteriorly to the right.

Recent Clinical Studies

In a 2023 publication, Basha *et al.* presented findings from a single-center retrospective cohort study [6]. Within this research, 17 subjects underwent computed tomography (CT)-guided trigeminal tractotomy/nucleotomy. Among these, therapeutic inefficacy was observed in six patients, with seven instances of failed cures. The median duration until the resurgence of pain was 5.6 months (IQR, 6.2). In another subset of 6 patients treated with caudalis DREZ, half reported efficacious pain mitigation lasting beyond a year, with a median pain recurrence time of 3.9 months (IQR, 29.53). Basha *et al.* surmised that the outcomes of the CT-oriented trigeminal tractotomy/nucleotomy exhibit variability, emphasizing the inherent challenges in managing trigeminal neuropathy pain.

Subsequent research by Tan *et al.* showed the clinical ramifications of CT-guided trigeminal tractotomy-nucleotomy [7]. They posited that the intervention, when administered under local anesthesia, presented tolerability issues stemming from the mandated cranial positioning in the conscious patient. Transitioning their approach, Tan *et al.* evaluated the efficacy and outcomes of this procedure in a cohort of 25 patients, totaling 31 interventions, all under general anesthesia. An impressive success rate of 74% (23/31) was documented. Remarkably, 50% and 40% of these procedures proffered pain alleviation spanning a minimum of 6 and 12 months, respectively, with a median pain relief duration of 153 days. Notably, transient and minor adverse events manifested in 6/31 procedures, constituting 19%. Intriguingly, a body mass index exceeding 25 emerged as a potential risk factor for suboptimal results (p=0.045). Conversely, heightened electrode ablation temperatures (p=0.033) and trajectories more medially aligned to the midsagittal plane (p=0.029) correlated with enhanced patient outcomes. Tan *et al.*'s overarching conclusion underscored the safety and efficacy of CT-guided trigeminal tractotomy-nucleotomy when performed under general anesthesia. Diverse findings have also been mirrored in other scholarly articles [9 - 10]. It is important to mention the paucity of microendoscopic tractotomy research, which shall be elaborated upon in subsequent sections [1, 11, 12].

Microendoscopic Trigeminal Nucleotractotomy

The first application of a percutaneous procedure on the trigeminal descending tract was described by Crue and associates in 1967. With the patient awake in the prone position, using a stereotactic frame and simple coordinates and electrophysiological control, and after a frustrating cisterna magna cisternography, a successful percutaneous radiofrequency lesion was made in the descending spinal trigeminal tract in a patient with facial pain caused by ethmoidal cancer, causing hypoalgesia in his ipsilateral forehead and occipital. Hitchcock, 1968, described the full stereotactic trigeminal tractotomy in a non-related work.

In 1970, a pioneering study reported the therapeutic outcomes of five oncogenic pain patients, one individual presenting with atypical facial discomfort, and another diagnosed with trigeminal neuralgia. By 1972, the nomenclature "trigeminal nucleosome" had been conferred upon the procedure by Schwarz. This advanced modality effectively mitigated complications that had plagued earlier open interventions. A graphical representation detailing the posterior dimensions of the inferior brainstem and the multitude of lesion sites fashioned during open trigeminal nucleotractotomy is provided in Fig. (**2**).

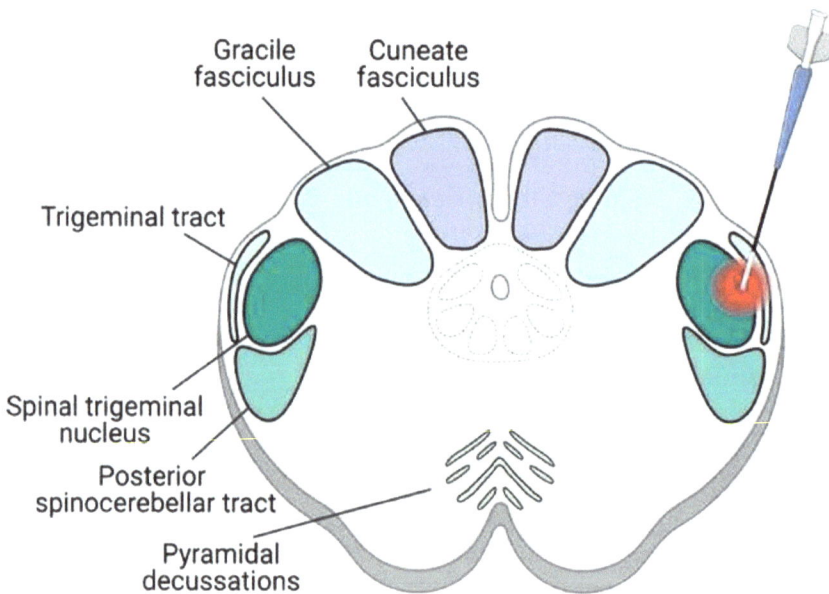

Fig. (2). Schematic representation of aspects of the lower brain stem, showing the multiple radiofrequency lesion sites during open trigeminal nucleotractotomy.

Our institutional protocol is rooted in the adaptation of the endoscopic tractotomy methodology delineated by Hitchcock and Teixeira, who have vividly characterized the pontine stereotactic trigeminal nucleotractotomy. In our clinic, the patient is positioned in a seated posture. Positive ventriculography or stereotomography is employed to demarcate the fourth ventricle (Fig. 3 and 4) occipito does not need to be bold, please change to regular font. The insertion of the endoscope is meticulously carried out between the occipito-atlantoaxial joint (C0-C1), with the fastigial line serving as an anatomical landmark. The strategic target lies at a distance of 5–10 mm from the median line, and 1 mm posterior to

6.6 mm anterior relative to the fourth ventricle's base. The vertical coordinates extend from 10.5 mm rostral to 1.2 mm caudal in reference to the fastigial line. Here, an electrode is maneuvered toward this locus. Impedance tracking is instrumental in ascertaining electrode contact with neural pathways and nuclei, while electrical stimulation discerns specific neural configurations. Notably, target point stimulation (<1 V; 5–100 Hz) induces ipsilateral facial tingling; stimulation of the trigeminal quintothalamic tract evokes contralateral facial tingling; stimulation of the trigeminal motor nucleus prompts ipsilateral masseter muscular contractions; stimulation of the facial nucleus triggers ipsilateral facial muscular contractions; and, vestibular nucleus stimulation yields an ipsilateral auditory hum. Following the meticulous positioning of the electrode, a radiofrequency lesion is sculpted, succeeded by an assessment of facial sensibility.

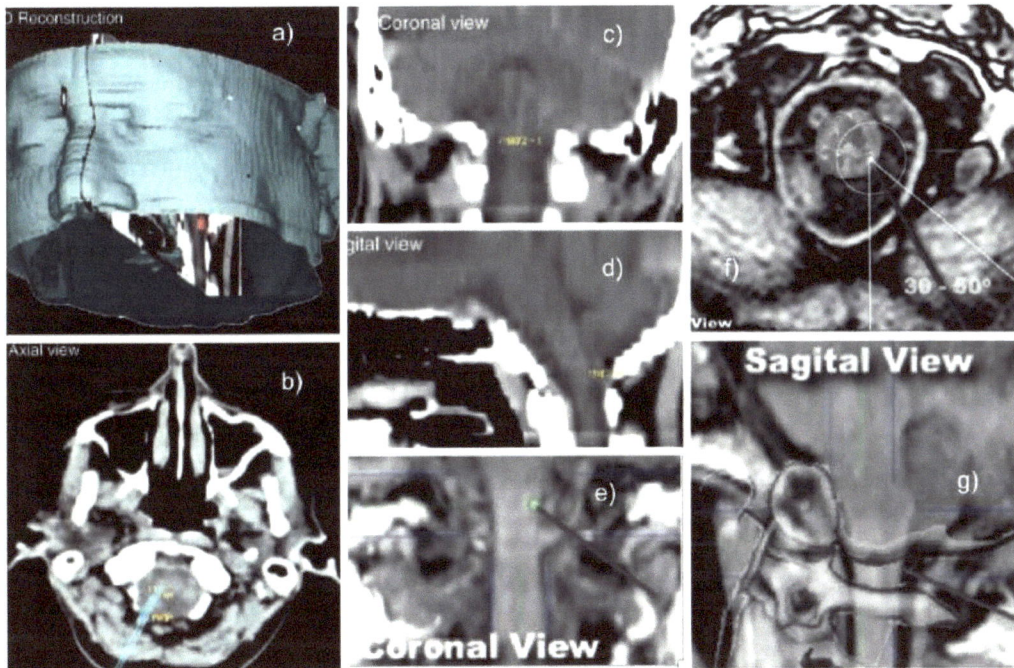

Fig. (3). Images show the endoscopy approach entering between the occipitocervical junction and the planned radiofrequency lesion sites during endoscopic trigeminal nucleotractotomy. Modified from: J Neurosurg. 2012 Feb;116(2):331-5.

DISCUSSION

The advent of Micro-Endoscopic Trigeminal Nucleotractotomy (MENT) has been recognized as a pioneering, minimally invasive modality tailored for the therapeutic management of Trigeminal Neuralgia (TN). This severe neuropathic facial pain disorder, characterized by episodic, sharp facial discomfort, is notorious for hampering mastication, speech and social interaction conversations. The ultimate therapeutic aim is to control this incapacitating pain, given its profound ramifications on patients' holistic well-being. Preliminary findings from our small cohort delineate the promising efficacy, safety, and feasibility of MENT as a contemporary microendoscopic intervention. A palpable diminution in pain intensity was witnessed post-MENT, substantiated by a downtrend in the Visual Analog Scale (VAS) scores; commencing from an average preoperative score of 8-10/10 to an average postoperative score of 2/10 at 4 weeks. This notable amelioration underscores MENT's potential to interrupt nociceptive pathways of the trigeminal nerve.

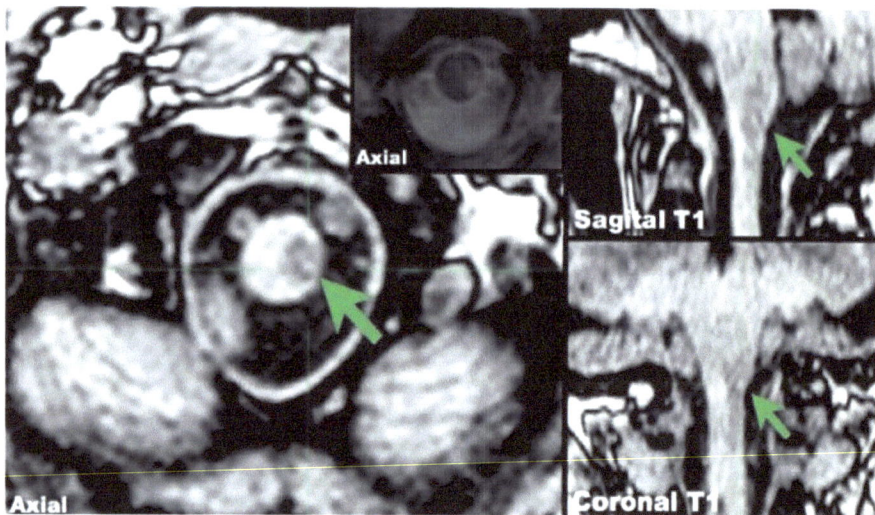

Fig. (4). The images show the postoperative MRI sequences which illustrate the lesion spot in the posterolateral aspects of the medulla, represented by a dot slightly hyperintense surrounded by hypointense edema in a larger. Modified from: J Neurosurg. 2012 Feb;116(2):331-5.

While the preliminary success of MENT is evident, its longevity in assuring sustained analgesia warrants meticulous scrutiny. A myriad of determinants, including judicious patient selection, precision in surgical technique, and TN's etiological roots, significantly modulate MENT outcomes. Ideal MENT candidates often grapple with relentless TN, impervious to standard therapeutic regimens. Discerning TN's etiology, be it idiopathic or secondary to vascular impingement, is pivotal, in influencing surgical prognosis. Surgical prowess, especially the exactitude in nucleotomy and tractotomy targeting within the trigeminal anatomical landscape, becomes indispensable. In our series, a nuanced microendoscopic methodology was employed, ensuring lesion precision and thorough ablation. Albeit devoid of any surgical mishaps in our cohort, expertise, and ascension on the learning trajectory cannot be neglected when dissecting the technique's clinical translatability. Potential sequelae, such as infections or neurosensory aberrations, though not observed, remain plausible. Rigorous patient stratification, impeccable surgical finesse, and robust training paradigms can attenuate complication probabilities. Delving deeper into the interaction between TN's pathogenesis and MENT's efficacy remains a research frontier.

Present studies, while illuminative, are not devoid of constraints. Their retrospective design, coupled with the confined sample and temporal follow-up, inflicts potential biases, particularly when juxtaposed against our extensive endoscopic expertise. This proficiency gradient is an often underestimated confounder in the MENT therapy. A clarion call for methodically designed, expansive, prospective investigations, augmented with extended monitoring and comparative cohorts, emerges to bolster the validity of MENT-associated clinical outcomes.

It is important to underscore that, while the data spans a limited temporal frame, TN's chronic trajectory necessitates protracted intervention strategies. Our findings corroborate with extant literature, exhibiting functional recuperation post-MENT in TN patients. A majority of our cohort demonstrated notable functional recovery, manifesting in improved masticatory, articulatory, and daily functional capacities. Such amelioration illustrates MENT's dual efficacy, alleviating not only pain but also rejuvenating functional prowess and overall life quality.

CONCLUSION

The therapeutical efficacy of Micro-Endoscopic Trigeminal Nucleotractotomy (MENT) results in marked analgesic relief and functional enhancement for individuals grappling with Trigeminal Neuralgia (TN). MENT, a paradigm of minimally invasive intervention for TN, synergistically amalgamates the merits of nucleotomy and tractotomy, further enriched by the granular visualization conferred by micro-endoscopy. Our clinical experience highlights the salient therapeutic benefits and safety profile of MENT in the TN therapeutic landscape. Notably, our observational cohort experienced no adverse events, a testament to our surgical team's expertise. To reinforce and expand upon our preliminary insights, future endeavors should include methodical, expansive prospective evaluations, bolstered with elongated patient monitoring; especially as MENT crystallizes as a standard institutionalized directive.

REFERENCES

[1]   Teixeira MJ, de Almeida FF, de Oliveira YSA, Fonoff ET. Microendoscopic stereotactic-guided percutaneous radiofrequency trigeminal nucleotractotomy. J Neurosurg 2012; 116(2): 331-5.

[http://dx.doi.org/10.3171/2011.8.JNS11618] [PMID: 21999320]

[2]   Pagni CA. CA P. Central pain and painful anesthesia. Prog Neurol Surg 1977; 8: 132-257.
[http://dx.doi.org/10.1159/000399868]

[3]   FWL K. The divisional organization of afferent fibers of the trigeminal nerve. Brain. J Neurosurg 1963; 86(72132)

[4]   Stewart WA, Stoops WL, Pillone PR, King RB. An electrophysiologic study of ascending pathways from nucleus caudalis of the spinal trigeminal nuclear complex. J Neurosurg 1964; 21(1): 35-48.
[http://dx.doi.org/10.3171/jns.1964.21.1.0035] [PMID: 14110357]

[5]   Weinberger LM. LM W. Experiences with intramedullary tractotomy. Arch Neurol Psychiatry 1942; 48(3): 355-81.
[http://dx.doi.org/10.1001/archneurpsyc.1942.02290090011001]

[6]   Basha AKMM, Simry HAM, Abdelbar AE, Sabry H, Raslan AM. Outcome of Surgical Treatments of Chronic Pain Caused by Trigeminal Neuropathy. World Neurosurg 2023; 170: e57-69.
[http://dx.doi.org/10.1016/j.wneu.2022.10.057] [PMID: 36273728]

[7]   Tan H, Ward E, Stedelin B, Raslan AM. Percutaneous CT-guided trigeminal tractotomy-nucleotomy under general anesthesia for intractable craniofacial pain. J Neurosurg 2022; •••: 1-9.
[http://dx.doi.org/10.3171/2022.10.JNS222144] [PMID: 36461818]

[8]   Kanpolat Y, Savas A, Batay F, Sinav A. Computed tomography-guided trigeminal tractotomy-nucleotomy in the management of vagoglossopharyngeal and geniculate neuralgias. Neurosurgery 1998; 43(3): 484-90.
[http://dx.doi.org/10.1097/00006123-199809000-00045] [PMID: 9733303]

[9]   Kanpolat Y, Kahilogullari G, Ugur HC, Elhan AH. Computed tomography-guided percutaneous trigeminal tractotomy-nucleotomy. Neurosurgery 2008; 63(1) (Suppl. 1): ONS147-53.
[PMID: 18728592]

[10]   Thompson EM, Burchiel KJ, Raslan AM. Percutaneous trigeminal tractotomy–nucleotomy with use of intraoperative computed tomography and general anesthesia: report of 2 cases. Neurosurg Focus 2013; 35(3)E5
[http://dx.doi.org/10.3171/2013.6.FOCUS13218] [PMID: 23991818]

[11]   Chen J, Sindou M. Vago-glossopharyngeal neuralgia: a literature review of neurosurgical experience. Acta Neurochir (Wien) 2015; 157(2): 311-21.
[http://dx.doi.org/10.1007/s00701-014-2302-7] [PMID: 25526720]

[12]   Blue R, Spadola M, McAree M, Kvint S, Lee JYK. Endoscopic Microvascular Decompression for Vagoglossopharyngeal Neuralgia. Cureus 2020; 12(12)e12353
[PMID: 33520548]

CHAPTER 3

Endonasal Endoscopic Approaches to the Sellar Region and the Anterior Fossa

Edgar G. Ordóñez-Rubiano[1], **Oscar Zorro**[1], **Nicolás Rincón Arias**[1], **Nadin J. Abdalá-Vargas**[1], **Javier G. Patiño-Gómez**[1] and **William Omar Contreras López**[2,*]

[1] *Department of Neurosurgery, Hospital de San José – Fundación Universitaria de Ciencias de la Salud, Los Mártires, Bogotá, Cundinamarca, Colombia*

[2] *Clínica Foscal Internacional, Autopista Floridablanca - Girón, Km 7, Floridablanca, Santander, Colombia*

Abstract: Endonasal endoscopic approaches have revolutionized surgical access to the sellar region and anterior fossa. These minimally invasive techniques utilize the natural nasal corridors to reach the target area, avoiding the need for external incisions. The endoscope provides excellent visualization and magnification, enabling precise surgical maneuvers. In this chapter, the authors describe the anatomical features for performing endoscopic endonasal approaches to the Sella and the anterior fossa. These approaches include the traditional endoscopic transsphenoidal approach to the Sella and extended endonasal approaches, including trans tuberculum, transplant, and transcribriform approaches. The most remarkable anatomical landmarks and surgical tenets are discussed. The anterior fossa houses critical structures like the anterior cranial base and the olfactory system. These structures can be approached for the resection of tumors, repair of cerebrospinal fluid leaks, and management of traumatic injuries. Endonasal endoscopic approaches offer reduced morbidity, shorter hospital stays, and faster recovery than traditional open approaches. Our clinical series shows that technological advancements and modern endoscopic surgical techniques further enhance the safety and efficacy of conventional transnasal methods, making them indispensable tools in the armamentarium of contemporary skull-base surgeons.

Keywords: Anterior fossa, Cribriform plate, Endonasal endoscopic, Endoscopic skull base surgery, Planum sphenoidale, Pituitary gland, Sellar region, Transsphenoidal, Tuberculum sellae.

---

* **Corresponding author William Omar Contreras López:** Clínica Foscal Internacional, Autopista Floridablanca - Girón, Km 7, Floridablanca, Santander, Colombia; Tel: +573112957003; E-mail: wcontreras127@unab.edu.co

Kai-Uwe Lewandrowski & William Omar Contreras López (Eds.)
All rights reserved-© 2024 Bentham Science Publishers

INTRODUCTION

Henry Schloffer described the first case of a transsphenoidal approach for resection of a hypophyseal tumor in 1907 [1]. Later, Harvey Cushing popularized this approach, modifying the original Schloffer technique [2, 3]. However, for decades mostly due to the limited light penetration in a narrow surgical corridor, Cushing's technique was replaced by complete transcranial procedures [4]. Guiot's introduction of the fluoroscope for intraoperative guidance, which was complemented by the use of the microscope by Hardy, contributed to the rebirth of this approach [5, 6]. Guiot also reported the first transsphenoidal surgery using an endoscope after endoscopic surgery was invented in the early 1800s [1]. In the mid-1960s, Storz, in collaboration with Hopkins, created the Storz-Hopkins endoscope, which contributed to the development of endoscopic technology. This new version brought optical improvements, better visualization, improved illumination, and provided a smaller and more flexible instrument [7]. One decade later, Apuzzo *et al.* [8], as well as Bushe and Halves [9] in Germany, began the description of combined microsurgical and endoscopic techniques for better visualization of skull base anatomical landmarks. Later, Jho and Carrau described their one-nasal fossa technique without using a nasal speculum, achieving a purely endonasal endoscopic approach (EEA) [10, 11]. Finally, during the late 1900s and early 2000s, new endoscopic schools began to appear, with several groups of neurosurgeons and otorhinolaryngologists investigating the surgical tenets, advantages, and limitations [12 - 17] of the technique. This chapter will focus on the anatomy and surgical features of the endoscopic endonasal approach (EEA) to the sella turcica and of its extended versions to the anterior skull base.

Endoscopic Endonasal Transsphenoidal Approach

Today, EEA represents the most widely used approach for sellar pathology. Most sellar and suprasellar tumors are accessed by opening the anterior aspect of the sella. Given the versatility of the endoscope and of endoscopic instruments, the manipulation of firm and soft tumors is feasible without the need to open the tuberculum sellae. If needed, the wide exposure of bony landmarks within the sphenoid sinus allows opening laterally to the anterior aspect of the cavernous sinus and the optic canal if going anteriorly. The traditional microscopic transsphenoidal approach was used for most pituitary adenomas for decades. Still, the advantages of the EEA, primarily improving magnification and visualization of critical structures and eliminating the need for brain retraction while minimizing manipulation of neurovascular structures, has promoted a trend towards minimally invasive endoscopic access [15, 18].

Endoscopic Anatomy & Surgical Technique

The wide intra-sphenoidal exposure begins with a straightforward approach from the nasal fossae. The nasal septum (pictured in the center of Fig. **1a**), the superior turbinate, and the choana are identified when entering the nares. At this point, the nasoseptal flap is normally harvested, if needed, for most of the extended approaches. A submucous transseptal approach is made. A resection of the vomer and the perpendicular plate of the ethmoid is performed. In some instances, these pieces of cartilage and bone are used to reconstruct the bony defect. Here, the sphenoid rostrum and keel are identified (Fig. **1b**) and drilled until the sphenoid sinus is opened. The intra-sphenoidal septum is resected. Then, the sella is observed, and the optic-carotid recesses (OCRs) are identified laterally on both sides (Fig. **1c**). Here, the anterior wall of the sella is drilled to expose the dura of the pituitary gland (Fig. **1d**). If needed, the bone is opened from the carotid protuberance of one side to the other. Most pituitary macroadenomas are resected through this approach, achieving a safe gross total resection (Fig. **2**).

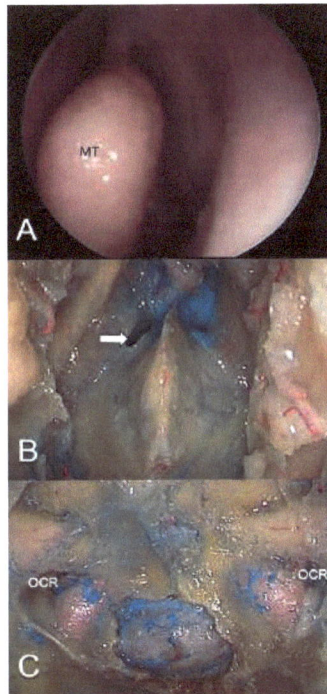

Fig. (1). Anatomy of the endoscopic endonasal approach. (**A**) The middle turbinate (MT) and the nasal septum are pictured. (**B**) The keel and the rostrum sphenoidale are observed, and the ostium of the right sphenoid sinus is marked with an arrow. (**C**) The sphenoid sinus is opened widely. The optic and the carotid protuberances are observed bilaterally. The optic-carotid recesses (OCR) are shown bilaterally.

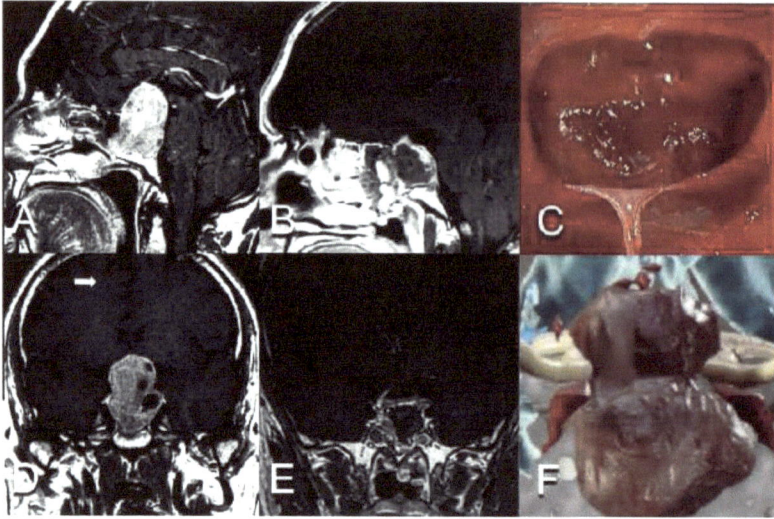

Fig. (2). Resection of a pituitary macroadenoma. (**A, D**) Preoperative enhanced T1 MRI demonstrating a large sellar and suprasellar macroadenoma. (**B, E**) Postoperative images demonstrate a near-total resection with a satisfactory decompression of the optic apparatus and preservation of the pituitary stalk and pituitary gland. (**C**) Endoscopic view of the resection cavity. (**F**) 3D reconstruction of the tumor and its relationship with the optic nerves and the internal carotid arteries bilaterally.

Endoscopic Transtuberculum Transplanum Approach

In the last two decades, the development and evolution of new endoscopes and new endoscopic instruments have allowed for increasingly safer manipulation of neurovascular structures. Using 30° and 45° scopes permits access to a long list of structures in the axial and coronal planes. Although the first transtuberculum transplant approaches were conducted using a microscope with the assistance of an endoscope [19], the extended EEA (EEEA) for a transtuberculum transplant corridor has been performed purely endoscopically by some groups, most notably by Kassam *et al.* in the early 2000s [12]. Unfortunately, given the low visualization quality of earlier endoscopes and many other limitations, including the surgical instruments and lack of expertise, this approach generated elevated rates of cerebrospinal fluid (CSF) leaks [20]. For the extended approach, most of the tumors treated through this corridor need a wide bony and dural opening [21, 22] (*e.g.*, tuberculum sellae meningiomas, craniopharyngiomas).

For most craniopharyngiomas, the best route remains the extended transtuberculum transplant approach (Fig. **3**) [14]. Despite this approach being reported for purely intrinsic thirdventricular craniopharyngiomas [23], other transcranial corridors have been proposed to be more feasible for a maximally safe resection [24].

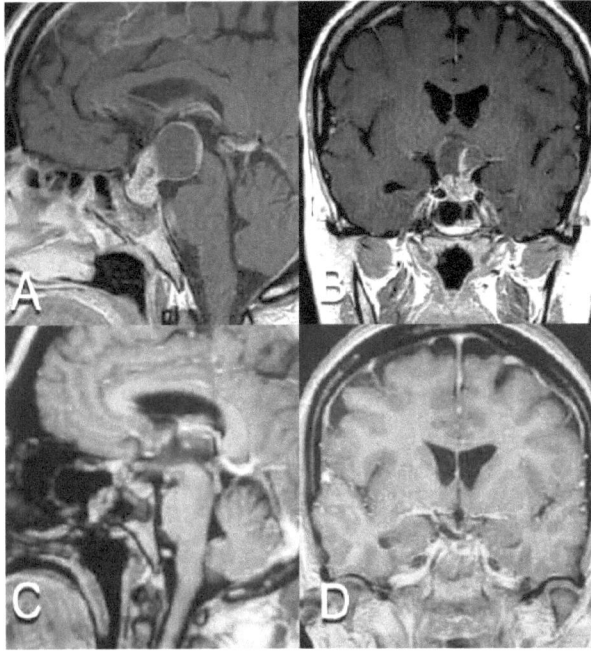

Fig. (3). Resection of a craniopharyngioma through an extended endonasal transtuberculum transplanum approach. (**A**, **B**) Preoperative enhanced T1 MRI showing a sellar and suprasellar tumor with heterogeneous enhancing with both solid and cystic components, extending into the third ventricle with a displacement of the optic apparatus. (**C**, **D**) Postoperative enhanced T1 MRI demonstrating a gross total resection of the tumor and decompression of the optic chiasm.

On the other hand, for tuberculum sellae meningiomas, the literature remains controversial [29 - 31]. The use of multiple endonasal [25] and transcranial, both endoscopic [26] and microscopic [25, 27], approaches were described for the resection of tuberculum sellae meningiomas [28]. Many limitations, including neurovascular encasement and the lateral extension of the tumor, as well as the higher risks of CSF leaking, remain essential considerations for patient and approach selection for resection.

After the anesthetics are administered, a lumbar drain is placed. The patient is supine, and a vascularized nasoseptal flap is raised and set aside for subsequent reconstruction. A wide sphenoidotomy and a posterior ethmoidectomy are done. The bone removal includes the top and the superior aspect of the anterior wall of the sella, the tuberculum sellae, and parts of the planum sphenoidale, as required according to the tumor size. The medial opticocarotid recesses constitute the lateral extent of bone resection (Table **1**).

Table 1. Advantages of endonasal endoscopic approaches.

Traditional Endoscopic Endonasal Approach - Provides a Direct and Wider View of the Surgical Field.
˙Allows for a more vertical angle of approach, which can be advantageous for accessing lesions located lower in the sellar region.
˙Is generally preferred for smaller tumors located in the midline of the sellar region.
˙Low risk of complications such as cerebrospinal fluid leaks and meningitis.
Endoscopic transtuberculum transplanum - Provides a horizontal angle of approach which can be advantageous for accessing lesions located higher in the sellar region.
˙Is a more suitable approach for larger tumors that extend more laterally,
Superiorly, or posteriorly into the third ventricle.
Endoscopic transethmoidal transcribiform - Provides a vertical angle of approach, which is ideal for accessing tumors located at the anterior cranial fossa.
˙Offers a direct and wide view of the surgical field, including the anterior cranial fossa and the sellar region.

The superior intercavernous sinus is identified, coagulated, and cut. The tumor is identified, internally debulked, and separated from adjacent neurovascular structures using sharp dissection. For craniopharyngiomas, all attempts are made to preserve the stalk if possible, and a sacrifice of the stalk is performed at the end of the process if necessary to achieve a complete resection. The superior hypophyseal arteries are preserved, and the branch to the stalk is sacrificed only if required for selected cases where the goal is to achieve a gross total resection. When treating a meningioma, all neurovascular structures, including the optic apparatus and the hypophyseal arteries, are preserved (Fig. **4**)—the closure changes according to the surgeon's preference and experience. In our institution, we perform a gasket-seal closure using a piece of bone or cartilage, and an onlay piece of autologous fascia lata larger than the bone defect is countersunk with a rigid buttress. Finally, this reconstruction is subsequently covered with a nasoseptal flap.

Endoscopic Transethmoidal Transcribiform Approach & Technique

The endoscopic transcribiform approach is limited anteriorly by the posterior wall of the frontal sinus; posteriorly, it is delimited by the posterior ethmoidal arteries and laterally by the lamina papyracea bilaterally (Table **2**). The most remarkable landmarks are the anterior and posterior ethmoidal arteries. In most cases, all the ethmoid is resected, and a Draft II sinusotomy is performed. This approach compromises the olfactory function and is limited only to selected cases like esthesioneuroblastomas (Fig. **5**), sinus carcinomas, and some olfactory groove meningiomas, among others.

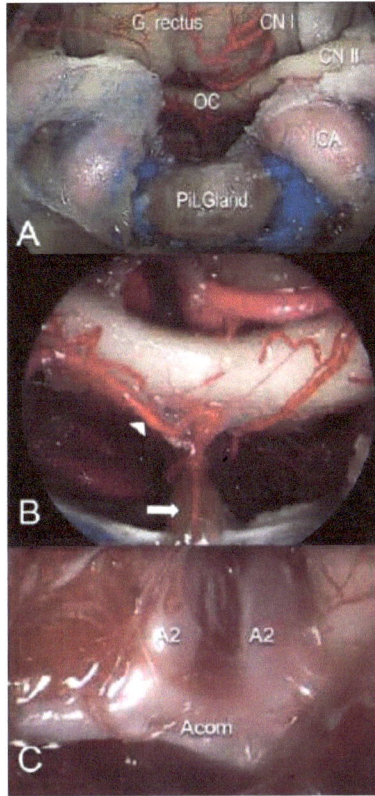

Fig. (4). Endoscopic anatomy of the endonasal transtuberculum transplanum approach. (**A**) Wide exposure of the sellar and anterior fossa components is demonstrated. In the midline, from anterior to posterior: the optic nerves – cranial nerve II (CN II), the optic chiasm (OC), the infundibulum, and the pituitary gland (Pit. Gland) are illustrated. Laterally the internal carotid artery (ICA), as well as the ophthalmic artery, are shown. An extended exposure to the cribriform plate was performed, allowing observation of the gyrus rectus (G. rectus) and the cranial nerve I (CN I) bilaterally. (**B**) A straightforward view of the suprasellar space is pictured. The optic chiasm and the pituitary stalk (arrow) are shown. The superior hypophyseal artery (arrowhead) and the optic and infundibular perforants are indicated. (**C**) An intraoperative endoscopic endonasal view of the anterior communicating complex is shown. The anterior communicating artery (Acom), as well as the A1 and A2 segments of the anterior cerebral arteries, are observed bilaterally, after the resection of a tuberculum sellae meningioma.

Table 2. Surgical corridors, landmarks, and limits of the endoscopic transethmoidal transcribiform and endoscopic transtuberculum transplanum approaches.

-	Endoscopic Transethmoidal Transcribiform Approach	Endoscopic Transtuberculum Transplanum Approach
Surgical corridor	- Complete ethmoid and frontal sinus. Draft II sinusotomy	- Posterior sphenoid and ethmoid
Anterior limit	- Posterior wall of the frontal sinus	- Posterior ethmoidal artery
Posterior limit	- Posterior ethmoidal arteries	- Sella

(Table 2) cont.....

-	Endoscopic Transethmoidal Transcribiform Approach	Endoscopic Transtuberculum Transplanum Approach
Lateral limit	- Lamina papyracea	- Optical canal - Paraclinoid segment aneurysms of the ICA
Anatomical landmarks	- Medial opticocarotid recesses - Optical canal	- Medial opticocarotid recesses - Optical canal

ICA: Internal carotid artery.

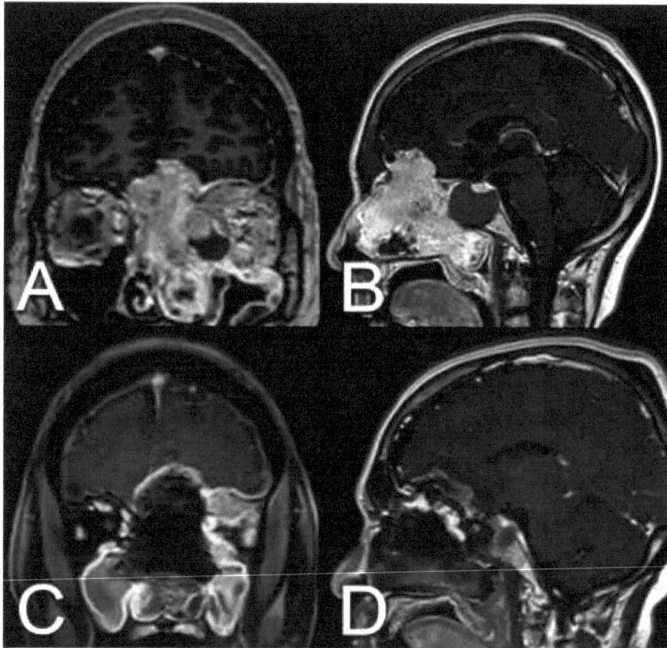

Fig. (5). Endoscopic transethmoidal transcribiform resection of an esthesioneuroblastoma. (**A, B**) Coronal and sagittal T1 post-contrast images demonstrate a large enhancing tumor occupying the complete endonasal space, extending into the nasopharynx, obstructing the sphenoid sinus, and entering the anterior fossa. (**C, D**) Postoperative enhanced MRI demonstrates a satisfactory resection with decompression of the breathing airway. A multilayer reconstruction is observed.

The uncinate process is identified, and the bunionectomy and infundibulotomy are performed. At this point, the ethmoidal bulla and the frontal recess are exposed. The bulla is entered, and the ethmoidectomy is completed to expose the fovea ethmoidal. The anterior ethmoidal artery is identified, coagulated, and cut (Fig. **6**). It is usually identified at the junction of the lamina papyracea and the frontal recess, delineating the anterior aspect of the ethmoidectomy. Middle turbinates are resected, and the lamina papyracea is exposed from anterior to posterior. In the posterior aspect of the ethmoid, at the lateral junction with the planum sphenoidale, the posterior ethmoidal arteries are exposed, coagulated, and cut.

Finally, the arteries are controlled and the bony ethmoidectomy is completed. The cribriform plate dura and the fovea ethmoidalis are exposed and removed to expose the rectus gyri.

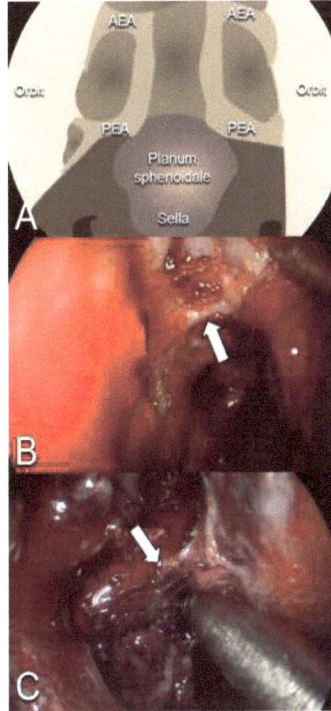

Fig. (6). Transethmoidal transcribiform approach. (**A**) A graphic illustration depicts the anatomical exposure of bony landmarks from below. The orbits, the anterior ethmoidal arteries (AEA), and the posterior ethmoidal arteries (PEA) are shown. (**B**) An intraoperative image illustrates the exposure of the right AEA (arrow) extending from the lamina papyracea to the ethmoid bone, which is compromised by a tumor. (**C**) An endonasal endoscopic view of the left PEA (arrow) is observed. The PEA extends from the posterior aspect of the left orbit to a vascularized tumor.

In our clinical series, we evaluated the efficacy and safety of EEA to the sella turcica and to the anterior skull base in the management of sellar pathologies our minimally invasive endoscopic EEA procedure that combines the principles of tumor resection and endoscopic access to minimize trauma and complications. We analyzed the outcomes in our small EEA series of patients with symptomatic lesions, including pain relief, functional improvement, and associated complications.

Our retrospective analysis was conducted on a consecutive series of patients diagnosed with sellar and anterior fossa pathologies who underwent EEA between 2018-2021. Patient demographics, preoperative diagnoses, clinical characteristics, surgical details, and postoperative outcomes were collected from medical records. Visual outcomes were assessed using postoperative visual fields. Postoperative MRI was performed for evaluation of radiological resection. Adverse events and complications related to the EEA procedure were also documented.

A total of 78 patients were included in the analysis. The mean age was 51.2 years, being 40 females. Patients presented with adenomas, craniopharyngiomas, esthesioneuroblastomas, and tuberculum sellae meningiomas. The main underlying cause of symptomatic pathology was optic apparatus compression. EEA was performed using an endoscope to visualize and access the sellar and anterior fossa content. Surgical techniques were standardized across the series. All patients presented no changes or improvement of visual function after surgical resection. A gross-total resection was achieved in 65% of the cases, a near-total resection in 20%, and partial resection in 15%. 2 patients (2.66%) presented CSF leaking, 1 patient (1,33%) required further hormone replacement due to new-onset endocrine deficit, and 2 patients (2.66%) presented non-neurosurgical complications after surgery including 1 patient (1,33%) with pneumonia and 1 patient (1,33%) with pulmonary embolism.

DISCUSSION

The endoscopic endonasal approach (EEA) to the sella turcica has revolutionized the field of skull base surgery. The sella turcica, a saddle-shaped bony structure located at the base of the skull, houses the pituitary gland and is a common site for the development of pituitary adenomas, craniopharyngiomas, and other sellar region pathologies. The EEA provides a minimally invasive alternative to traditional open approaches for accessing and treating these lesions. The sella turcica, which houses the pituitary gland, has been one of the primary targets for EEA. Pituitary adenomas, which are commonly found in this region, can be effectively managed using this approach. The ability to access and remove these tumors through the nasal corridor provides several advantages. Firstly, it allows for complete tumor resection while preserving normal pituitary gland function. Secondly, it eliminates the need for a transcranial approach, reducing the risk of brain injury and associated complications. Studies have consistently demonstrated high rates of surgical success, ranging from 80% to 95%, in achieving complete or near-complete resection of pituitary adenomas using EEA. In addition to pituitary adenomas, other sellar region pathologies, such as craniopharyngiomas and Rathke's cleft cysts, can also be effectively managed using EEA.

Facial incisions or craniotomies are no longer necessary. The ability to approach these lesions through the nasal corridor provides excellent visualization and access to the entire sellar region, facilitating safe and complete tumor resection.

The endoscope also provides a magnified view, enabling surgeons to identify and spare the functional parts of the pituitary gland during tumor resection. By carefully dissecting the nasal passages, surgeons can gain access to the anterior skull base, achieving optimal tumor resection while preserving critical neurovascular structures. In addition to the improved surgical outcomes, EEA for pituitary adenomas offers the advantage of preserving normal pituitary gland function. This preservation of pituitary function minimizes the risk of postoperative hormonal deficiencies and contributes to improved patient quality of life. Furthermore, EEA allows for precise reconstruction of the skull base using graft materials to prevent postoperative cerebrospinal fluid leaks, a common complication in skull base surgery. Improved surgical techniques and advancements in reconstructive materials have significantly reduced the incidence of such complications, further enhancing the outcomes of EEA.

While EEA offers several advantages, it is not without limitations. The technique requires a high level of surgical expertise and familiarity with nasal anatomy. Surgeons must have a comprehensive understanding of the sinonasal passages, the skull base anatomy, and the relationships of the critical structures in order to navigate through these complex regions safely. In addition, the learning curve for EEA can be steep, and it often requires a multidisciplinary team approach involving neurosurgeons and otolaryngologists experienced in endoscopic skull base surgery. However, with proper training and experience, these challenges can be overcome, leading to successful outcomes.

CONCLUSIONS

EEA and the extended versions to access the anterior skull base have been improving over time, and indications have been restricted to selected cases to avoid complications, especially CSF leaking. Excellent knowledge of endoscopic skull base anatomy for each corridor and the learning curve for reconstructive techniques are key points for good performance in endoscopic endonasal skull base surgery. Proper exposure to the identification of bony and neurovascular landmarks is paramount for satisfactory surgical results. Extracranial and intracranial components of each corridor are fundamental for maximizing structural and functional outcomes.

REFERENCES

[1]   Wang AJ, Zaidi HA, Laws ED Jr. History of endonasal skull base surgery. J Neurosurg Sci 2016; 60(4): 441-53.
[PMID: 27273318]

[2]   Cushing H III. III. Partial Hypophysectomy for Acromegaly: With Remarks on the Function of the Hypophysis. Ann Surg 1909; 50(6): 1002-17.
[http://dx.doi.org/10.1097/00000658-190912000-00003] [PMID: 17862444]

[3] Cushing H. The Weir Mitchell lecture: surgical experiences with pituitary disorders. J Am Med Assoc 1914; LXIII(18): 1515-25.
[http://dx.doi.org/10.1001/jama.1914.02570180001001]

[4] Liu JK, Das K, Weiss MH, Laws ER Jr, Couldwell WT. The history and evolution of transsphenoidal surgery. J Neurosurg 2001; 95(6): 1083-96.
[http://dx.doi.org/10.3171/jns.2001.95.6.1083] [PMID: 11765830]

[5] Hardy J, Wigser SM. Trans-sphenoidal surgery of pituitary fossa tumors with televised radiofluoroscopic control. J Neurosurg 1965; 23(6): 612-9.
[http://dx.doi.org/10.3171/jns.1965.23.6.0612] [PMID: 5861144]

[6] Hardy J. [Surgery of the pituitary gland, using the trans-sphenoidal approach. Comparative study of 2 technical methods]. Union Med Can 1967; 96(6): 702-12.
[PMID: 5630039]

[7] Linder TE, Simmen D, Stool SE. Revolutionary inventions in the 20th century. The history of endoscopy. Arch Otolaryngol Head Neck Surg 1997; 123(11): 1161-3.
[http://dx.doi.org/10.1001/archotol.1997.01900110011001] [PMID: 9366694]

[8] Apuzzo MLJ, Heifetz MD, Weiss MH, Kurze T. Neurosurgical endoscopy using the side-viewing telescope. J Neurosurg 1977; 46(3): 398-400.
[http://dx.doi.org/10.3171/jns.1977.46.3.0398] [PMID: 839267]

[9] Bushe KA, Halves E. Modified technique in transsphenoidal operations of pituitary adenomas. Technical note. Acta Neurochir (Wien) 1978; 41(1-3): 163-75.
[http://dx.doi.org/10.1007/BF01809147] [PMID: 665329]

[10] Carrau RL, Jho HD, Ko Y. Transnasal-transsphenoidal endoscopic surgery of the pituitary gland. Laryngoscope 1996; 106(7): 914-8.
[http://dx.doi.org/10.1097/00005537-199607000-00025] [PMID: 8667994]

[11] Jho HD, Carrau RL. Endoscopic endonasal transsphenoidal surgery: experience with 50 patients. J Neurosurg 1997; 87(1): 44-51.
[http://dx.doi.org/10.3171/jns.1997.87.1.0044] [PMID: 9202264]

[12] Kassam A, Snyderman CH, Mintz A, Gardner P, Carrau RL. Expanded endonasal approach: the rostrocaudal axis. Part I. Crista galli to the sella turcica. Neurosurg Focus 2005; 19(1): 1-12.
[http://dx.doi.org/10.3171/foc.2005.19.1.4] [PMID: 16078817]

[13] Schwartz TH, Stieg PE, Anand VK. Endoscopic transsphenoidal pituitary surgery with intraoperative magnetic resonance imaging. Neurosurgery 2006; 58(1) (Suppl.): ONS44-51.
[PMID: 16479628]

[14] Ordóñez-Rubiano EG, Forbes JA, Morgenstern PF, *et al.* Preserve or sacrifice the stalk? Endocrinological outcomes, extent of resection, and recurrence rates following endoscopic endonasal resection of craniopharyngiomas. J Neurosurg 2018; 1-9.
[PMID: 30497145]

[15] Cappabianca P, Alfieri A, Stefano T, Buonamassa S, Enrico D. Instruments for endoscopic endonasal transsphenoidal surgery. Neurosurgery 1999; 45(2): 392-5.
[http://dx.doi.org/10.1097/00006123-199908000-00041] [PMID: 10449087]

[16] Frank G, Pasquini E, Mazzatenta D. Extended transsphenoidal approach. J Neurosurg 2001; 95(5): 917-8.
[PMID: 11702890]

[17] Zoli M, Milanese L, Bonfatti R, *et al.* Clival chordomas: considerations after 16 years of endoscopic endonasal surgery. J Neurosurg 2018; 128(2): 329-38.
[http://dx.doi.org/10.3171/2016.11.JNS162082] [PMID: 28409727]

[18] Prevedello DM, Ebner FH, de Lara D, Filho LD, Otto BA, Carrau RL. Extracapsular dissection

technique with the Cotton Swab for pituitary adenomas through an endoscopic endonasal approach – How I do it. Acta Neurochir (Wien) 2013; 155(9): 1629-32.
[http://dx.doi.org/10.1007/s00701-013-1766-1] [PMID: 23793961]

[19]   Kaptain GJ, Vincent DA, Sheehan JP, Laws ER Jr. Transsphenoidal approaches for the extracapsular resection of midline suprasellar and anterior cranial base lesions. Neurosurgery 2008; 62(6) (Suppl. 3): SHC1264-71.
[http://dx.doi.org/10.1227/01.NEU.0000333791.29091.83] [PMID: 18695546]

[20]   Zanation AM, Carrau RL, Snyderman CH, *et al.* Nasoseptal flap reconstruction of high flow intraoperative cerebral spinal fluid leaks during endoscopic skull base surgery. Am J Rhinol Allergy 2009; 23(5): 518-21.
[http://dx.doi.org/10.2500/ajra.2009.23.3378] [PMID: 19807986]

[21]   Gardner PA, Prevedello DM, Kassam AB, Snyderman CH, Carrau RL, Mintz AH. The evolution of the endonasal approach for craniopharyngiomas. J Neurosurg 2008; 108(5): 1043-7.
[http://dx.doi.org/10.3171/JNS/2008/108/5/1043] [PMID: 18447729]

[22]   Conger AR, Lucas J, Zada G, Schwartz TH, Cohen-Gadol AA. Endoscopic extended transsphenoidal resection of craniopharyngiomas: nuances of neurosurgical technique. Neurosurg Focus 2014; 37(4)E10
[http://dx.doi.org/10.3171/2014.7.FOCUS14364] [PMID: 25270129]

[23]   Forbes JA, Ordóñez-Rubiano EG, Tomasiewicz HC, *et al.* Endonasal endoscopic transsphenoidal resection of intrinsic third ventricular craniopharyngioma: surgical results. J Neurosurg 2018; 1-11.
[PMID: 30497140]

[24]   Al-Mefty O, Ayoubi S, Kadri PA. The petrosal approach for the total removal of giant retrochiasmatic craniopharyngiomas in children. J Neurosurg 2007; 106(2) (Suppl.): 87-92.
[PMID: 17330531]

[25]   Li Y, Zhang C, Su J, *et al.* Individualized surgical treatment of giant tuberculum sellae meningioma: Unilateral subfrontal approach vs. endoscopic transsphenoidal approach. Front Surg 2022; 9990646
[http://dx.doi.org/10.3389/fsurg.2022.990646] [PMID: 36743895]

[26]   Sasaki T, Morisako H, Ikegami M, Wardhana DW, Fernandez-Miranda JC, Goto T. Endoscopic supraorbital eyebrow approach for medium-size tuberculum sellae meningiomas; a cadaveric stepwise dissection, technical nuances and surgical outcomes. World Neurosurg 2023; 176: e40-8.
[http://dx.doi.org/10.1016/j.wneu.2023.03.063]

[27]   Caklili M, Emengen A, Yilmaz E, *et al.* Endoscopic Endonasal Approach Limitations and Evolutions for Tuberculum Sellae Meningiomas: Data from Single-Center Experience of Sixty Patients. Turk Neurosurg 2023; 33(2): 272-82.
[PMID: 36622191]

[28]   Jimenez AE, Harrison Snyder M, Rabinovich EP, *et al.* Comparison and evolution of transcranial versus endoscopic endonasal approaches for suprasellar Meningiomas: A systematic review. J Clin Neurosci 2022; 99: 302-10.
[http://dx.doi.org/10.1016/j.jocn.2022.03.029] [PMID: 35325729]

CHAPTER 4

Pathophysiology of Myelomeningocele and Modern Surgical Treatment

William Omar Contreras López[1,*], Jezid Miranda Quintero[2], Cristóbal Abello Munárriz[3], Guido Parra Anaya[4], Kai-Uwe Lewandrowski[5,6,7], Juan David Hernandez[8] and Miguel Parra Saavedra[4,9]

[1] *Clínica Foscal Internacional, Autopista Floridablanca - Girón, Km 7, Floridablanca, Santander, Colombia*

[2] *Departamento de Ginecología, Facultad de Medicina, Grupo de Investigación en Cuidado Intensivo y Obstetricia (GRICIO), Universidad de Cartagena, Cartagena de Indias, Colombia*

[3] *Centro Médico CEDIUL, CEDIFETAL, Barranquilla, Colombia*

[4] *Departamento de Ginecología y Obstetricia, División de Medicina Maternofetal, Clínica General del Norte, Barranquilla, Colombia*

[5] *Center for Advanced Spine Care of Southern Arizona and Surgical Institute of Tucson, Tucson, AZ, USA*

[6] *Departmemt of Orthopaedics, Fundación Universitaria Sanitas, Bogotá, D.C., Colombia*

[7] *Department of Neurosurgery in the Video-Endoscopic Postgraduate Program at the Universidade Federal do Estado do Rio de Janeiro - UNIRIO, Rio de Janeiro, Brazil*

[8] *Sociedad Colombiana de Anestesiología, Departamento Anestesiología, Clínica General del Norte, Barranquilla, Colombia*

[9] *Universidad Simón Bolívar, Barranquilla, Colombia*

Abstract: Myelomeningocele (MMC) is the most relevant clinical variant of spina bifida - a birth defect resulting in an open vertebral column. The failure of the lumbosacral neural tube to close during embryonic development may compromise the spinal cord *in utero* due to exposure to amniotic fluid and irritation by the uterine wall. Resulting neurological deficits may vary depending on the spinal level involved. Most neural tube defects are diagnosed in the second trimester by ultrasound. Early prenatal diagnosis allows *in-utero* repair to diminish neurological deficits and the need for postnatal ventricular shunting. In this chapter, the authors present a brief review of the pathophysiology of fetal MMC and the various repair options, and their associated clinical outcomes. Clinical studies suggest improved short-term neurological outcomes with percutaneous minimally invasive and intrauterine fetoscopic techniques using endoscopes compared with an open prenatal or postnatal repair. The main limitations of these modern techniques are preterm premature rupture of membranes (PPROM) and

---

[*] **Corresponding author William Omar Contreras López:** Clínica Foscal Internacional, Autopista Floridablanca - Girón, Km 7, Floridablanca, Santander, Colombia; Tel: +573112957003; E-mail: wcontreras127@unab.edu.co

Kai-Uwe Lewandrowski & William Omar Contreras López (Eds.)

dehiscence or leakage at the MMC repair. Additional benefits may include a lower risk of preterm labor, reduced need for postnatal revisions, and improved newborn maturity with higher gestational age. Fetoscopy may also offer better management of the membranes and primary closure of uterine port sites. The long-term cognitive, behavioral, and functional outcomes of fetoscopic MMC repair have yet to be determined. While cesarean section may be required for delivery in subsequent pregnancies after traditional open prenatal MMC repair to avoid uterine rupture, fetoscopic methods with externalization of the uterus by maternal laparotomy may allow spontaneous vaginal delivery at term.

Keywords: Fetoscopy, Lumbosacral neural tube, Myelomeningocele, Neurological deficits, Spina bifida.

INTRODUCTION

Spina bifida is a birth defect in which the vertebral column is open, commonly compromising the spinal cord. Myelomeningocele (MMC) is the most relevant clinical variant, which is characterized by the lumbosacral neural tube remaining open during embryonic development. *In-utero* exposure degenerates neural tissue, resulting in a neurological deficit that varies according to the level of injury. Prenatal diagnosis is achieved by ultrasound in the second trimester of pregnancy, allowing for a repair *in utero* to prevent neurological deficits. Fetal MMC repair has been associated with improved short-term neurological outcomes compared with postnatal repair. In recent years, these techniques have made it possible to reduce the neurological impact and the quality of life of the affected individuals. Currently, the establishment of a standardized surgical technique is being debated. These standards are beneficial to ensure the best results for patients and their families. This chapter aims to summarize the main aspects concerning the pathophysiology of myelomeningocele, its prenatal diagnosis, and the principal current therapeutic options.

Pathophysiology

Genetic and non-genetic factors contribute to neural tube defects [1]. The genetic risk has been estimated at 60-70% based on the relative rate of involvement in twins [2]. Less than 10% of neural tube defects are syndromic, with expressions of chromosomal disorders such as trisomy 13 or 18. The majority are non-syndromic and occur sporadically. Accumulating evidence in recent years has shown a model of multifactorial origin for nonsyndromic neural tube defects, which includes multiple genes and non-genetic factors [1]. The fact that the majority of fetuses and newborns affected with anencephaly are female suggests a sex-associated genetic factor or an epigenetic component in anencephaly [3].

Folate deficiency is one of the most important non-genetic MMC risk factors. Factors that escalate the probability of spina bifida are iterated in Table **1**.

Table 1. Risk factors for neural tube defects.

Maternal Nutritional Factors	Other Maternal Factors	Environmental Factors
Use of alcohol	Smoking	Air pollution
Use of caffeine	Hyperthermia in the first trimester	Disinfectant contaminants in drinking water
Low intake of folates	Low socioeconomic level	Components related to nitrates
High glycemic index	Maternal diseases and infections	Organic solvents
Low methionine intake	Insulin-dependent pregestational diabetes	Pesticides
Low AFP levels	Pre-gestational obesity	Polycyl aromatic hydrocarbons
Low serum levels of vitamin B12	Psychological stress	-
Low levels of vitamin C	Use of valproic acid	-
Low zinc levels	-	-

At the core of MMC pathophysiology lies an embryonic aberration wherein the neural tube in the spinal domain of the embryo remains unsealed. Such a defect culminates in the sustained exposure of the neural tube to the amniotic milieu [1]. Vertebrates undergo two distinct stages in the formation of the medullary canal; the primary neurulation and subsequent canalization. In Homo sapiens, the onset of primary neurulation is marked at the juncture between the prospective brain stem and cervical spine approximately 22 days subsequent to fertilization. From this nexus, there is a bidirectional closure of the neural tube, both cranially towards the brain stem and caudally towards the spine. By the 24th gestational day, the cranial sealing culminates at the rostral neuropore. Contrarily, spinal closure persists over an extended period, methodically constituting the neuraxis until its termination at the caudal neuropore around the 26th day, achieving closure proximate to the sacrum [1, 4].

Neural tube defects (NTD) can occur due to failure of any of the aforementioned processes and are typically open defects, due to failure of the neuronal folds at the level of the dorsal midline [1]. The most severe NTD is craniorachischisis, which is characterized by the combination of anencephaly (absence of the brain and cranial vault, without skin covering) with a contiguous bony defect of the spine (also without meninges or sac covering the neural tissue – rachischisis or myeloschisis). In the case of this defect, closure fails to initiate on day 22. If the embryo successfully initiates closure, but cranial neurulation subsequently fails, anencephaly results. Conversely, failure of spinal neurulation after the initiation of closure generates spina bifida, with the axial level varying depending on the affected wave of closure [1]. As gestation progresses, the exposed spinal cord begins to become hemorrhagic, neurons die from amniotic fluid toxicity, axonal connections are disrupted, and the function is lost [1]. Therefore, neurological dysfunction is considered a "double-crush" process. First, a defective closure of the neural tube occurs, which is then followed by secondary neurodegeneration in utero due to mechanical trauma from the uterine wall and chemical damage *via* the amniotic fluid.

Folate deficiency is associated with MMC. It is estimated that approximately 70% of MMC can be prevented by increasing available maternal folic acid levels in the preconception period until the seventh week of pregnancy, at which time neural tube closure is complete [5]. The recommended dose is 400 micrograms, starting at least 3 months before conception [6]. The association with maternal obesity is very high and is particularly more related to spina bifida than to anencephaly [7]. It is important to emphasize that spina bifida related to maternal obesity may not be effectively prevented with folic acid [8]; as it may be related to incorrect glucose metabolism, oxidative stress, and metabolic syndrome [9].

Associated Neurological Alterations

MMC is associated with brain malformations and hydrocephalus. The principal brain defect involves Chiari II-associated abnormalities affecting the brain stem, which impacts nearly all such fetuses in the absence of antenatal repair [1, 10, 11]. The anomaly correlates with cerebellar evolution within a confined posterior fossa, engendering cerebellar protrusion *via* the foramen magnum and concomitant perturbations in the brain stem, cisterna magna, and both third and fourth ventricles [12]. To elucidate further, a structural reconfiguration of the cerebellum occurs, wherein its anterior aspect is augmented and, conversely, the posterior and inferior facets are attenuated; however, the cerebellar white matter, or medullary body, remains unchanged [13]. It has been observed that cerebellar volume diminution is more pronounced in instances of thoracic lesions as juxtaposed with lumbar or sacral afflictions, however, a universal reduction is discerned across all lesion categories [14]. Moreover, a staggering 65% of MMC patients exhibit a deformation in the brainstem, characterized by a posteriorly oriented tectal aberration that invaginates into the cerebellum [1]. In a significant 70% of the patient population, the cord manifests as protracted and convoluted at the spinomedullary juncture [15]. Conclusively, the cisterna magna is notably absent, and there is a diminution in the dimensions of the third and fourth ventricles.

Radiological evaluations indicate that the basal ganglia and subcortical architectures in spina bifida-afflicted individuals are preserved in their normative state [15]. Macrostructural investigations have revealed a contraction in the hippocampal volume [16]. A range of one-third to half of the pediatric MMC demographic exhibit dysgenesis of the corpus callosum, predominantly impacting either the splenium coupled with the posterior body, or the rostrum [17]. Hydrocephalus emerges as an additional sequela of MMC, instigated chiefly by an impediment in cerebrospinal fluid flow at the fourth ventricle's ambit; however, other influential elements include stenosis of the Sylvian aqueduct, alterations in venous hemodynamics, and ependymal denudation. Finally, a cortical reorganization is also evidenced in fetuses with MMC, with enlarged frontal regions, while a reduction in volume has been described in the posterior cortical regions [17]. Studies using diffusion imaging of white matter structures show that the organizing tracts connecting the anterior and posterior brain regions are consistently reduced in individuals with MMC [18, 19]. These reductions in frontal volume compared to posterior regions have been associated with a decrease in intelligence, and in cognitive and motor functions [20, 21].

MMC also causes motor dysfunction, the severity of which depends on the level of the injury, with the probability of walking decreasing the higher the injury. Patients with injuries at the level of L2 or above are typically wheelchair dependent; injuries between L3 and L5 require some type of ambulatory assistance; and injuries at S1 or below allow for unassisted walking. Musculoskeletal manifestations include kyphosis, scoliosis, hip dislocations, contractures, and clubfoot; with all of the these alterations producing great disability for the individual.

Diagnosis and Screening

In the 1970s, prenatal identification of MMC was made possible thanks to the identification of high concentrations of alpha-fetoprotein in the amniotic fluid, and later in the serum of women with affected pregnancies [1]. Currently, with the expanded use of ultrasonography in obstetrics and the introduction of second trimester ultrasound to screen for morphological alterations, antenatal identification of the defect has increased drastically [1]. Statistics indicate that the detection of fetuses with MMC in experienced prenatal diagnosis centers is as high as 90-98%. However, there is a clear inequality in prenatal diagnosis rates according to the level of economic development of the country [22 - 24].

In prenatal diagnostics, fetal ultrasonography is the preeminent tool for the identification of spina bifida. Utilizing ultrasound, the fetal spine can be meticulously scrutinized in sagittal, axial, and coronal orientations as early as the inaugural trimester; thereby furnishing anatomical visualization to discern the morphology, topography, and extent of the aberration. Ultrasound assessments are viable during the embryonic phase (11-14 weeks) as well as during the fetal development phase (18-22 weeks). While specific intracranial sonographic indicators have been delineated, there are also relevant findings on the fetal vertebrae. Ultrasound implicates intracranial involvement when a conspicuous decrement in the biparietal diameter exists relative to the gestational timeline, or when ventriculomegaly is evident [25].

In the history of medical imaging, the quintessential lemon and banana signs were articulated by Nicolaides *et al.* in the 20th century's penultimate decade [26, 27]. The "lemon sign" refers to the attenuation of the frontal bone's convexity, culminating in a flattened aspect, and is discernible in virtually all MMC-afflicted fetuses from week 16 to 24 (Refer to Fig. **1A**). Subsequent to the 24th week, this sign is observable in only 30-50% of the affected cohort [28]. Contrarily, the "banana sign" is emblematic of the cerebellar contour, postulated to arise from cerebellar traction subsequent to cerebral tissue herniation (Chiari II malformation; as illustrated in Fig. **1B**). This sign becomes perceptible from the 14th week onwards [29, 30]. It is noteworthy that at advanced gestational ages, ultrasonographic discernment of the cerebellum not possible in roughly 80% of affected cases, rendering the banana sign unhelpful as a diagnostic metric at these advanced junctures [30, 31]. The efficacy of ultrasonography in detecting cranial markers indicative of spina bifida is cataloged in Table **2**.

Table 2. Ultrasound detection rate of spina bifida cranial markers.

-	Ultrasonic Abnormality			-
Study	**Lemon Sign**	**Banana Sign**	**Ventriculomegaly**	**Microcephaly**
Nicolaides *et al.* [28]	100% (n=54)	95% (n=21)	62% (n=70)	86% (n=66)
Campbell *et al.* [27]	100% (n=26)	95% (n=26)	65% (n=26)	54% (n=26)
Nyberg *et al.* [32]	93% (n=14)	NR	NR	NR
Thiagarajah *et al.* [29]	100% (n=16)	100% (n=16)	69% (n=16)	63% (n=16)
Van den Hof *et al.* [31]	98% (n=107)	96% (n=107)	NR	NR
Bahlmann *et al.* [30]	88.6% (n=588)	97% (n=588)	46% (n=588)	70% (n=588)

The lemon and banana signs have high specificity, sensitivity, and positive predictive values. Other associated ultrasonographic signs include hydrocephalus and microcephaly. For the identification of the defect in the fetal spine, the main form of identification is found in the sagittal plane, particularly if the lesion is associated with meningocele or myelomeningocele, or when the cystic lesion extends ostensibly over the circulating skin (Fig. **2**). The presence of neural tissue within the sac can be detected by ultrasound. In addition to spina bifida, associated spinal abnormalities such as kyphoscoliosis can also be detected by ultrasound [1].

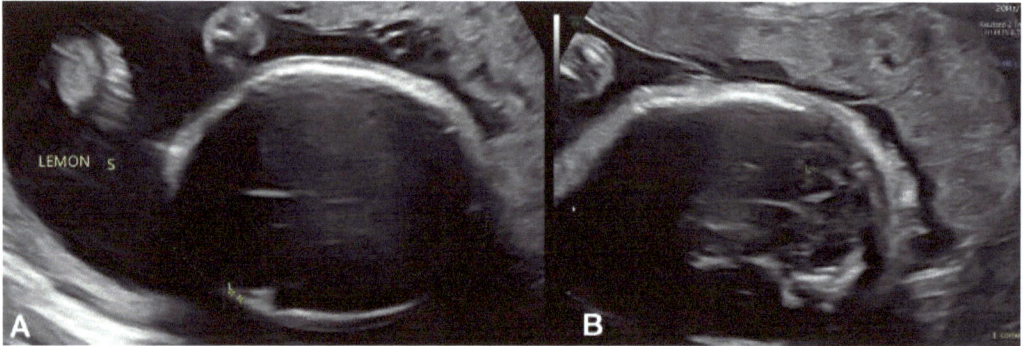

Fig. (1). Ultrasound diagnosis of spina bifida with classic intracranial ultrasound signs in axial section of a 26-week-old fetus. **A)** The lemon sign is described as the loss of the convex shape of the frontal bones, with flattening, and is present in almost all fetuses with MMC between weeks 16 and 24. **B)** The banana sign refers to the shape of the cerebellum, and is believed to be due to traction of the cerebellum after herniation of brain tissue. In this section of the posterior fossa, obliteration of the fourth ventricle and cisterna magna with anterior bulging of the cerebellum is observed. The association of the banana sign with Arnold's Chiari type II malformation is common.

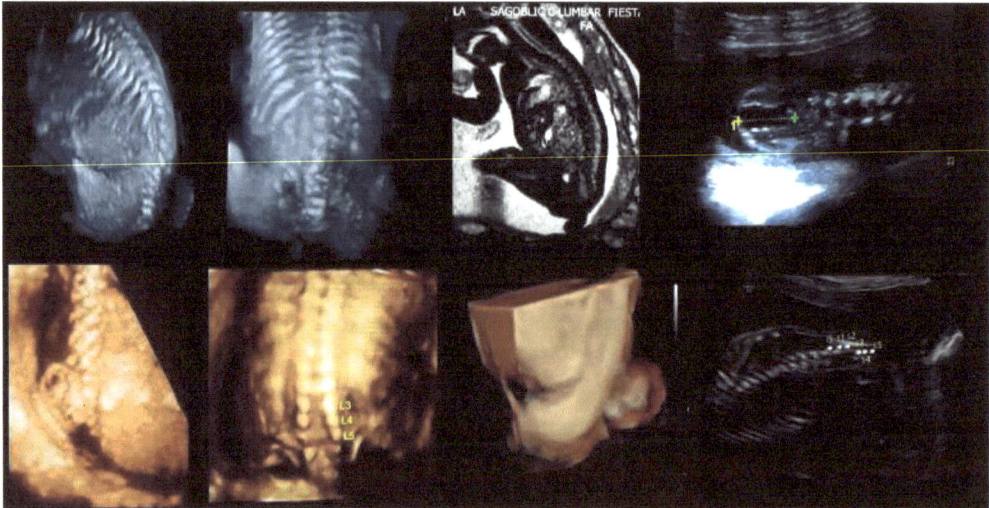

Fig. (2). A set of diagnostic images of patients with a cystic saccular appearance in the lower lumbar spine that protrudes due to a defect in posterior fusion of bone elements. The third image from left to right above is an intrauterine magnetic resonance image, where the closure defect of the neural tube at the sacral level is also visible.

Contemporary Treatment

The "dual-insult theory," dictates that neural structures, upon their exposure to amniotic fluid and coupled with persistent intrauterine adversities, undergo ancillary detriments as gestation unfolds [1]. The rationale behind performing intrauterine surgery to correct MMC is that the damage progresses during pregnancy [1, 33]. Women considering surgery in utero should complete a full prenatal study that includes obstetric evaluation, screening for chromosomal and genetic syndromes, ultrasound of the fetus to assess lower limb function, identification of additional defects, and determination of the level of spinal injury [1]. The open technique includes a maternal laparotomy, in which a hysterotomy of approximately 6-8 centimeters is performed, large enough to expose the lesion. Defect closure follows a standard procedure similar to postnatal closure. The cyst membrane is removed, the meninges that are in contact with the skin and soft tissue are mobilized, and the neural placode is separated from the surrounding tissue and removed, to be repositioned in the spinal canal. If possible, the dura is identified, aligned with the placode, and closed in the midline. Finally, the skin is closed to complete the repair [1].

The first successful *in-utero* repair was reported in 1998 [33] and the success of *in-utero* repair emerged in the literature in 1998 [34]. Subsequently, various institutions ventured into implementing the intervention despite the absence of unequivocal evidence supporting its advantage over postnatal interventions [35, 36]. To bridge this evidentiary gap, a meticulously designed prospective randomized clinical trial dubbed the "Management of Myelomeningocele Study" (MOMS), was initiated in 2003. This investigation aimed to compare maternal and fetal repercussions of MMC repair conducted between 19 to 25 gestational weeks with the conventional postnatal reparative approach [37].

The study's two primary facets included: 1) an array of fetal or neonatal determinants, notably mortality or the necessity for ventriculoperitoneal shunt placement within the first year of life, and 2) an aggregate score from the Bayley Scales of Infant Development II, combined with motor proficiency assessments performed 30 months post-partum. A comprehensive analysis began, however following 8 years of meticulous scrutiny involving 183 out of the planned 200 patients, the project prematurely terminated further patient enrolment. This early closure occurred due to ethical considerations, as preliminary findings indicated the pronounced efficacy of in utero intervention in substantially curtailing the necessity for shunt implementation. By the children's first birthday, the rate of ventriculoperitoneal shunt requirement was only 40% for the intrauterine intervention cohort, in stark contrast to the 82% observed in the postnatal counterpart. Further advantages were observed in enhanced neuromotor functions at 30 months, evidenced by an increased percentage of infants demonstrating ambulatory capabilities [37]. Complementarily, the incidence of brainstem herniations was conspicuously attenuated in the cohort who received fetal surgical intervention compared to their postnatal counterparts.

In the open modality employed in the MOMS, the fetal spinal defect is accessed *via* a laparotomy, followed by uterine exteriorization and subsequent hysterotomy. This procedural choice has been linked to increased maternal and fetal disadvantages; which include a heightened susceptibility to uterine rupture, a predisposition for cesarean section both in the present gestation and in subsequent ones, an escalated rate of preterm deliveries, and augmented perinatal mortality rates in subsequent pregnancies [38, 39]. Moreover, anomalies in the closure of the hysterotomy were evident in a significant 35% of cases, with 11% of cases manifesting partial to complete dehiscence [38]. Predominant complications in the prenatal repair cohort included chorioamniotic membrane detachment, early rupture of membranes, oligohydramnios, placental abruption, pulmonary edema, and transfusion requisites during parturition [38, 40]. While the precise etiologies elevating membrane rupture in the open modality for prenatal MMC repair remain unclear, recent empirical evidence suggests that the risk of preterm premature rupture of membranes (PPROM) stands at an alarming 60% when interventions occur between 20 and 21 weeks, as compared to 0% at precisely 25 6/7 weeks [41]. An ancillary consideration regarding the open methodology concerns the reproductive implications for the female patient, rendering it an essential consideration during familial counselling for this therapeutic avenue [42]. Postnatal outcome evaluations for subsequent pregnancies underscored a gestational attrition rate of 13%, alongside increased incidence for uterine dehiscence (17.3%), uterine rupture (9.65%), and stillbirths, (approximately 4%) [40].

Intrauterine Endoscopic Repair

Subsequent scrutiny of the "Management of Myelomeningocele Study" (MOMS) revealed obstetric outcomes, which suggested that the elevated incidences of premature rupture of membranes (30.7%), preterm deliveries, and additional obstetric difficulties could conceivably be attenuated through a fetoscopic approach to MMC repair. While the initial endeavors at antenatal MMC amelioration adopted an endoscopic trajectory, the technical impediments of the era resulted in its relegation, ushering in a pervasive reliance on the open surgical modality [43].

The resurrection of the fetoscopic modality for in utero spina bifida repair was inspired by the intent to minimize maternal adverse effects, and concomitant fetal and neonatal risks associated with open hysterotomy, while concurrently conserving the neurologic advantages provided to the neonate. Presently, the medical fraternity acknowledges two distinct minimally invasive methodologies:

1) The percutaneous approach [44-48], and 2) A fetoscopic variant entailing an externalized uterus [49-52].

Belfort *et al.*, representing the Texas Children's Fetal Center, championed a distinct fetoscopic technique that aimed to reduce the negative effects associated with both the open fetal and percutaneous fetoscopic MMC repair paradigms [51]. In contrast to methodologies employed by Kohl or Pedreira *et al.*, their intervention involved accessing the uterine chamber *via* maternal laparotomy and conducting the procedure *via* two 4-mm uterine ports. Following this, the membranes were anchored to the uterine wall using sutures, with the uterine port sites predominantly sutured using absorbable materials. Their meticulous approach, which encompassed a single-layer closure over the spinal cord without employing a patch, yielded a laudable 100% fetal and neonatal survival rate. Remarkably, the gestational age at birth under 37 weeks was 36%, a figure significantly lower than any hitherto reported cohort for fetal MMC repair [44]. This investigation stands as a milestone in demonstrating the feasibility of vaginal delivery (50%) post fetal MMC repair [49, 53].

In response to the considerable incidence rate of cerebrospinal fluid fistulas (25%) in comparison to the MOMS data, these researchers introduced a refined technique. This encompassed a tri-layer closure integrating a bovine collagen patch, a myofascial layer, and a cutaneous closure. This refinement achieved the complete eradication of CSF leaks and a notable decrement in postnatal interventions, such as ventriculoperitoneal shunts or ventriculostomies, for hydrocephalus [50].

In a bid to harmonize and refine the fetoscopic MMC repair modality, the International Consortium for the Study of Fetoscopic MMC Repair was incepted. This platform was devised to congregate diverse groups, fostering a transparent and symbiotic collaboration. A subsequent comparison of 300 cases utilizing fetoscopy (165 *via* the percutaneous method and 135 with the externalized uterus technique) was disseminated. The treatise reported congruent prenatal and 12-month postnatal outcomes between the open and fetoscopic modalities. Intriguingly, the fetoscopic approach proffered the additional benefit of enabling vaginal delivery, without the risks associated with uterine scar dehiscence (Table **3**) [54].

Table 3. Comparison of MOMs study clinical results with the open and minimally invasive fetoscopic techniques described.

Data	MOMs Study	Fetoscopy	P-Value
Gestational age at the time of surgery (weeks)	23.6 (±1.4)	26.16 (±1.6)	<0.01
Technique type	-	-	-
Hysterotomy	78 (100)	0	<0.01
Percutaneous	-	165 (55)	<0.01
Exteriorized uterus with laparotomy	-	135 (45)	<0.01
Surgery duration (minutes)	204 (72-458)	78.5 (54 – 106)	-
Fetal bradycardia during surgery requiring resuscitation	8 (10.3)	5 (1.7)	0.001
Placental abruption	5 (6.4)	25/280 (8.9)	0.64
Chorioamniotic membranes	20 (25.6)	72/190 (37.9)	0.06
Premature rupture of membranes	36 (46.2)	153/280 (54.6%)	0.2
Gestational age at birth (weeks)	34.1 (±3.1)	34.3 (±3.6)	0.63
Birth by caesarean section	78 (100)	192/280 (68.6)	<0.01
Hysterotomy status at the time of cesarean section	-	-	-
Intact, healed	49/76 (64.5)	162/162 (100)	<0.01
Slimmed down	19/76 (25)	0/162 (0)	<0.01
Dehisced area	7/76 (9.2)	0/162 (0)	<0.01
Dehiscence at the level of the spinal repair site	10/77 (13)	56/279 (20.1)	-
Motor function compared to a higher anatomical level	-	-	-
≥ two levels better	20/62 (32.3)	98/257 (38.1)	0.46
1 level better	7/62 (11.3)	63/257 (24.5)	<0.01
Similar	14/62 (21)	49/257 (19.1)	0.59
1 level worse	13/62 (21)	35/257 (13.6)	0.16
≥ two levels worse	8/62 (12.9)	12/257 (4.7)	0.03

Data are presented as n (%) or mean ± standard deviation.

It is imperative to underscore the fact that such outcomes are attainable solely within the ambit of an encompassing programmatic structure. This necessitates the integration of a neonatal intensive care unit in tandem with specialized neonatology services. Equally key is the establishment of a multidisciplinary spina bifida consortium, encompassing expertise from pediatric neurosurgery, urology, orthopedics, physical therapy, occupational therapy, and social work, among other specialized cohorts. Such an assembly is crucial to holistically address the myriad physical, psychological, and societal requisites of these patient demographics. The salience of continuous skill enhancement for the collective team, leveraging varied simulation paradigms, remains paramount for ensuring the technical prowess and resultant success of the surgical interventions (Fig. **3**).

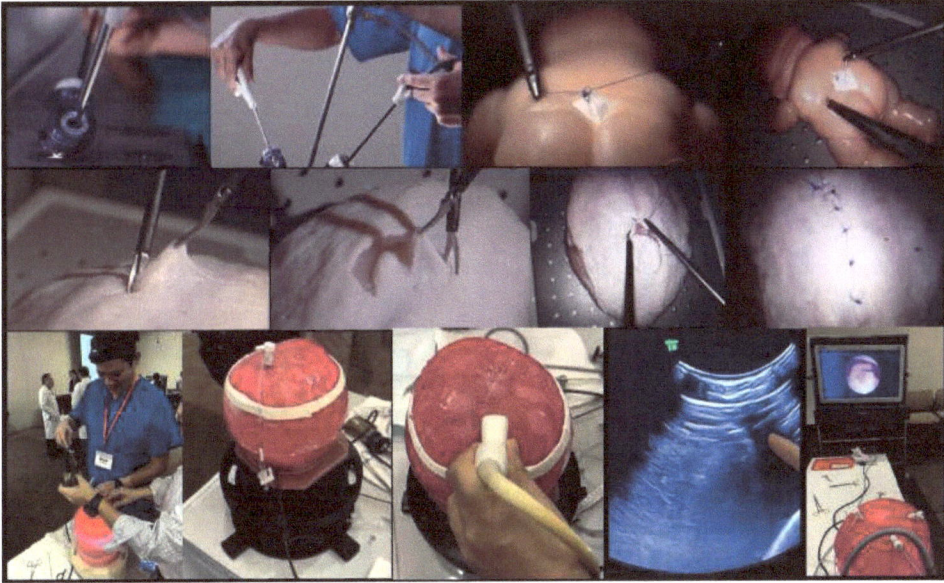

Fig. (3). Training to master the learning curve with the technique is extremely important. It consists of several stages. First, trainees undergo in-depth training at laparoscopy stations with models using dummies that simulate the MMC defect. The second phase includes training using chicken breasts, which are similar to the brittle skin and muscle of a 26-week fetus. The third phase includes training in simulation models that include CO2 inflated placenta, intraoperative ultrasound, and a myelomeningocele model shown in the lower panel (Training Model of the Texas Children 's Hospital, USA).

CONCLUSION

To date, the main limitations of fetoscopic percutaneous MMC repair are preterm premature rupture of membranes (PPROM) and dehiscence or leakage at the MMC repair site that require postnatal care. Minimally invasive and endosopic percutaneous fetoscopic approaches to MMC repair may offer a better alternative to the open approach if the technique can be further optimized to lower the risk of preterm labor, PPROM, and the need for postnatal revisions of the repair. Gestational age at birth improves with better management of the membranes and primary closure of uterine port sites, as seen in fetoscopic MMC repair achieved *via* maternal laparotomy. The long-term cognitive, behavioral, and functional outcomes of fetoscopic MMC repair have yet to be reported and compared to the gold standard of open fetal MMC repair. After open fetal surgery, a caesarean section is required for delivery in subsequent pregnancies because of the possibility of uterine rupture. According to the recently published results on more than 300 cases of fetoscopic MMC repair with externalization of the uterus by maternal laparotomy proposed by Belfort *et al.*, spontaneous vaginal delivery at term is possible; and this is the technique used at our center.

REFERENCES

[1]   Copp AJ, Adzick NS, Chitty LS, Fletcher JM, Holmbeck GN, Shaw GM. Spina bifida. Nat Rev Dis Primers 2015; 1(1): 15007.
[http://dx.doi.org/10.1038/nrdp.2015.7] [PMID: 27189655]

[2]   Carter CO, Evans K. Spina bifida and anencephalus in greater London. J Med Genet 1973; 10(3): 209-34.
[http://dx.doi.org/10.1136/jmg.10.3.209] [PMID: 4590246]

[3]   Juriloff DM, Harris MJ. Hypothesis: The female excess in cranial neural tube defects reflects an epigenetic drag of the inactivating x chromosome on the molecular mechanisms of neural fold elevation. Birth Defects Res A Clin Mol Teratol 2012; 94(10): 849-55.
[http://dx.doi.org/10.1002/bdra.23036] [PMID: 22753363]

[4]   Müller F, O'Rahilly R. The development of the human brain, the closure of the caudal neuropore, and the beginning of secondary neurulation at stage 12. Anat Embryol (Berl) 1987; 176(4): 413-30.
[http://dx.doi.org/10.1007/BF00310083] [PMID: 3688450]

[5]   Bevilacqua NS, Pedreira DAL. Fetoscopy for meningomyelocele repair: past, present and future. Einstein (Sao Paulo) 2015; 13(2): 283-9.
[http://dx.doi.org/10.1590/S1679-45082015RW3032] [PMID: 26154549]

[6]   Lumley J, Watson L, Watson M, Bower C. Periconceptional supplementation with folate and/or multivitamins for preventing neural tube defects. Cochrane Database Syst Rev 2001; (3): CD001056
[PMID: 11686974]

[7]   Stothard KJ, Tennant PWG, Bell R, Rankin J. Maternal overweight and obesity and the risk of congenital anomalies: a systematic review and meta-analysis. JAMA 2009; 301(6): 636-50.
[http://dx.doi.org/10.1001/jama.2009.113] [PMID: 19211471]

[8]   Parker SE, Yazdy MM, Tinker SC, Mitchell AA, Werler MM. The impact of folic acid intake on the association among diabetes mellitus, obesity, and spina bifida. Am J Obstet Gynecol 2013; 209(3): 239.e1-8.
[http://dx.doi.org/10.1016/j.ajog.2013.05.047] [PMID: 23711668]

[9]   Carmichael SL, Rasmussen SA, Shaw GM. Prepregnancy obesity: A complex risk factor for selected birth defects. Birth Defects Res A Clin Mol Teratol 2010; 88(10): 804-10.
[http://dx.doi.org/10.1002/bdra.20679] [PMID: 20973050]

[10]   Stevenson KL. Chiari Type II malformation: past, present, and future. Neurosurg Focus 2004; 16(2): 1-7.
[http://dx.doi.org/10.3171/foc.2004.16.2.6] [PMID: 15209488]

[11]   Yamashiro KJ, Galganski LA, Hirose S. Fetal myelomeningocele repair. Semin Pediatr Surg 2019; 28(4)150823
[http://dx.doi.org/10.1053/j.sempedsurg.2019.07.006] [PMID: 31451171]

[12]   McLone DG, Knepper PA. The cause of Chiari II malformation: a unified theory. Pediatr Neurosurg 1989; 15(1): 1-12.
[http://dx.doi.org/10.1159/000120432] [PMID: 2699756]

[13]   Juranek J, Dennis M, Cirino PT, El-Messidi L, Fletcher JM. The cerebellum in children with spina bifida and Chiari II malformation: Quantitative volumetrics by region. Cerebellum 2010; 9(2): 240-8.
[http://dx.doi.org/10.1007/s12311-010-0157-x] [PMID: 20143197]

[14]   Fletcher JM, Copeland K, Frederick JA, et al. Spinal lesion level in spina bifida: a source of neural and cognitive heterogeneity. J Neurosurg 2005; 102(3) (Suppl.): 268-79.
[PMID: 15881750]

[15]   Ware AL, Juranek J, Williams VJ, Cirino PT, Dennis M, Fletcher JM. Anatomical and diffusion MRI of deep gray matter in pediatric spina bifida. Neuroimage Clin 2014; 5: 120-7.
[http://dx.doi.org/10.1016/j.nicl.2014.05.012] [PMID: 25057465]

[16]   Treble-Barna A, Juranek J, Stuebing KK, Cirino PT, Dennis M, Fletcher JM. Prospective and episodic memory in relation to hippocampal volume in adults with spina bifida myelomeningocele. Neuropsychology 2015; 29(1): 92-101.
[http://dx.doi.org/10.1037/neu0000111] [PMID: 25068670]

[17]   Crawley JT, Hasan K, Hannay HJ, Dennis M, Jockell C, Fletcher JM. Structure, integrity, and function of the hypoplastic corpus callosum in spina bifida myelomeningocele. Brain Connect 2014; 4(8): 608-18.
[http://dx.doi.org/10.1089/brain.2014.0237] [PMID: 25014561]

[18]   Juranek J, Fletcher JM, Hasan KM, *et al.* Neocortical reorganization in spina bifida. Neuroimage 2008; 40(4): 1516-22.
[http://dx.doi.org/10.1016/j.neuroimage.2008.01.043] [PMID: 18337124]

[19]   Hasan KM, Eluvathingal TJ, Kramer LA, Ewing-Cobbs L, Dennis M, Fletcher JM. White matter microstructural abnormalities in children with spina bifida myelomeningocele and hydrocephalus: A diffusion tensor tractography study of the association pathways. J Magn Reson Imaging 2008; 27(4): 700-9.
[http://dx.doi.org/10.1002/jmri.21297] [PMID: 18302204]

[20]   Ou X, Glasier CM, Snow JH. Diffusion tensor imaging evaluation of white matter in adolescents with myelomeningocele and Chiari II malformation. Pediatr Radiol 2011; 41(11): 1407-15.
[http://dx.doi.org/10.1007/s00247-011-2180-6] [PMID: 21725712]

[21]   Hannay HJ, Walker A, Dennis M, Kramer L, Blaser S, Fletcher JM. Auditory interhemispheric transfer in relation to patterns of partial agenesis and hypoplasia of the corpus callosum in spina bifida meningomyelocele. J Int Neuropsychol Soc 2008; 14(5): 771-81.
[http://dx.doi.org/10.1017/S1355617708080958] [PMID: 18764972]

[22]   Treble A, Juranek J, Stuebing KK, Dennis M, Fletcher JM. Functional significance of atypical cortical organization in spina bifida myelomeningocele: relations of cortical thickness and gyrification with IQ and fine motor dexterity. Cereb Cortex 2013; 23(10): 2357-69.
[http://dx.doi.org/10.1093/cercor/bhs226] [PMID: 22875857]

[23]   Chitty LS. Ultrasound screening for fetal abnormalities. Prenat Diagn 1995; 15(13): 1241-57.
[http://dx.doi.org/10.1002/pd.1970151306] [PMID: 8710765]

[24]   Roberts T, Henderson J, Mugford M, Bricker L, Neilson J, Garcia J. Antenatal ultrasound screening for fetal abnormalities: a systematic review of studies of cost and cost effectiveness. BJOG 2002; 109(1): 44-56.
[http://dx.doi.org/10.1111/j.1471-0528.2002.00223.x] [PMID: 11843373]

[25]   Romosan G, Henriksson E, Rylander A, Valentin L. Diagnostic performance of routine ultrasound screening for fetal abnormalities in an unselected Swedish population in 2000–2005. Ultrasound Obstet Gynecol 2009; 34(5): 526-33.
[http://dx.doi.org/10.1002/uog.6446] [PMID: 19688769]

[26]   Biggio JR Jr, Owen J, Wenstrom KD, Oakes WJ. Can prenatal ultrasound findings predict ambulatory status in fetuses with open spina bifida? Am J Obstet Gynecol 2001; 185(5): 1016-20.
[http://dx.doi.org/10.1067/mob.2001.117676] [PMID: 11717624]

[27]   Campbell J, Gilbert WM, Nicolaides KH, Campbell S. Ultrasound screening for spina bifida: cranial and cerebellar signs in a high-risk population. Obstet Gynecol 1987; 70(2): 247-50.
[PMID: 3299184]

[28]   Nicolaides KH, Gabbe SG, Campbell S, Guidetti R. Ultrasound screening for spina bifida: cranial and cerebellar signs. Lancet 1986; 328(8498): 72-4.
[http://dx.doi.org/10.1016/S0140-6736(86)91610-7] [PMID: 2425202]

[29]   Thiagarajah S, Henke J, Hogge WA, Abbitt PL, Breeden N, Ferguson JE. Early diagnosis of spina bifida: the value of cranial ultrasound markers. Obstet Gynecol 1990; 76(1): 54-7.

[PMID: 2193270]

[30]   Bahlmann F, Reinhard I, Schramm T, *et al.* Cranial and cerebral signs in the diagnosis of spina bifida between 18 and 22 weeks of gestation: a German multicentre study. Prenat Diagn 2015; 35(3): 228-35.
[http://dx.doi.org/10.1002/pd.4524] [PMID: 25346419]

[31]   Van den Hof MC, Nicolaides KH, Campbell J, Campbell S. Evaluation of the lemon and banana signs in one hundred thirty fetuses with open spina bifida. Am J Obstet Gynecol 1990; 162(2): 322-7.
[http://dx.doi.org/10.1016/0002-9378(90)90378-K] [PMID: 2178424]

[32]   Nyberg DA, Mack LA, Hirsch J, Mahony BS. Abnormalities of fetal cranial contour in sonographic detection of spina bifida: evaluation of the "lemon" sign. Radiology 1988; 167(2): 387-92.
[http://dx.doi.org/10.1148/radiology.167.2.3282259] [PMID: 3282259]

[33]   Adzick NS. Fetal surgery for myelomeningocele: trials and tribulations. J Pediatr Surg 2012; 47(2): 273-81.
[http://dx.doi.org/10.1016/j.jpedsurg.2011.11.021] [PMID: 22325376]

[34]   Adzick NS, Sutton LN, Crombleholme TM, Flake AW. Successful fetal surgery for spina bifida. Lancet 1998; 352(9141): 1675-6.
[http://dx.doi.org/10.1016/S0140-6736(98)00070-1] [PMID: 9853442]

[35]   Sutton LN, Adzick NS, Bilaniuk LT, Johnson MP, Crombleholme TM, Flake AW. Improvement in hindbrain herniation demonstrated by serial fetal magnetic resonance imaging following fetal surgery for myelomeningocele. JAMA 1999; 282(19): 1826-31.
[http://dx.doi.org/10.1001/jama.282.19.1826] [PMID: 10573273]

[36]   Tulipan N, Hernanz-Schulman M, Bruner JP. Reduced hindbrain herniation after intrauterine myelomeningocele repair: A report of four cases. Pediatr Neurosurg 1998; 29(5): 274-8.
[http://dx.doi.org/10.1159/000028735] [PMID: 9917546]

[37]   Adzick NS, Thom EA, Spong CY, *et al.* A randomized trial of prenatal versus postnatal repair of myelomeningocele. N Engl J Med 2011; 364(11): 993-1004.
[http://dx.doi.org/10.1056/NEJMoa1014379] [PMID: 21306277]

[38]   Johnson MP, Bennett KA, Rand L, Burrows PK, Thom EA, Howell LJ, *et al.* The Management of Myelomeningocele Study: obstetrical outcomes and risk factors for obstetrical complications following prenatal surgery. Am J Obstet Gynecol 2016; 215(6): e1-9.
[http://dx.doi.org/10.1016/j.ajog.2016.07.052]

[39]   Johnson MP, Sutton LN, Rintoul N, *et al.* Fetal myelomeningocele repair: short-term clinical outcomes. Am J Obstet Gynecol 2003; 189(2): 482-7.
[http://dx.doi.org/10.1067/S0002-9378(03)00295-3] [PMID: 14520222]

[40]   Goodnight WH, Bahtiyar O, Bennett KA, Emery SP, Lillegard JB, Fisher A, *et al.* Subsequent pregnancy outcomes after open maternal-fetal surgery for myelomeningocele. Am J Obstet Gynecol 2019; 220(5): e1-7.
[http://dx.doi.org/10.1016/j.ajog.2019.03.008]

[41]   Soni S, Moldenhauer JS, Spinner SS, *et al.* Chorioamniotic membrane separation and preterm premature rupture of membranes complicating in utero myelomeningocele repair. Am J Obstet Gynecol 2016; 214(5): 647.e1-7.
[http://dx.doi.org/10.1016/j.ajog.2015.12.003] [PMID: 26692177]

[42]   Danzer E, Joyeux L, Flake AW, Deprest J. Fetal surgical intervention for myelomeningocele: lessons learned, outcomes, and future implications. Dev Med Child Neurol 2020; 62(4): 417-25.
[http://dx.doi.org/10.1111/dmcn.14429] [PMID: 31840814]

[43]   Bruner JP, Tulipan NE, Richards WO. Endoscopic coverage of fetal open myelomeningocele in utero. Am J Obstet Gynecol 1997; 176(1): 256-7.
[http://dx.doi.org/10.1016/S0002-9378(97)80050-6] [PMID: 9024126]

[44]   Degenhardt J, Schürg R, Winarno A, *et al.* Percutaneous minimal☐access fetoscopic surgery for spina

bifida aperta. Part II : maternal management and outcome. Ultrasound Obstet Gynecol 2014; 44(5): 525-31.
[http://dx.doi.org/10.1002/uog.13389] [PMID: 24753062]

[45]   Graf K, Kohl T, Neubauer BA, *et al.* Percutaneous minimally invasive fetoscopic surgery for spina bifida aperta. Part III: neurosurgical intervention in the first postnatal year. Ultrasound Obstet Gynecol 2016; 47(2): 158-61.
[http://dx.doi.org/10.1002/uog.14937] [PMID: 26138563]

[46]   Kohl T. Percutaneous minimally invasive fetoscopic surgery for spina bifida aperta. Part I: surgical technique and perioperative outcome. Ultrasound Obstet Gynecol 2014; 44(5): 515-24.
[http://dx.doi.org/10.1002/uog.13430] [PMID: 24891102]

[47]   Lapa Pedreira DA, Acacio GL, Gonçalves RT, *et al.* Percutaneous fetoscopic closure of large open spina bifida using a bilaminar skin substitute. Ultrasound Obstet Gynecol 2018; 52(4): 458-66.
[http://dx.doi.org/10.1002/uog.19001] [PMID: 29314321]

[48]   Pedreira DAL, Reece EA, Chmait RH, Kontopoulos EV, Quintero RA. Fetoscopic repair of spina bifida: safer and better? Ultrasound Obstet Gynecol 2016; 48(2): 141-7.
[http://dx.doi.org/10.1002/uog.15987] [PMID: 27273812]

[49]   Belfort MA, Whitehead WE, Shamshirsaz AA, *et al.* Fetoscopic Open Neural Tube Defect Repair. Obstet Gynecol 2017; 129(4): 734-43.
[http://dx.doi.org/10.1097/AOG.0000000000001941] [PMID: 28277363]

[50]   Belfort MA, Whitehead WE, Shamshirsaz AA, *et al.* Comparison of two fetoscopic open neural tube defect repair techniques: single☐ *vs* three☐layer closure. Ultrasound Obstet Gynecol 2020; 56(4): 532-40.
[http://dx.doi.org/10.1002/uog.21915] [PMID: 31709658]

[51]   Belfort MA, Whitehead WE, Shamshirsaz AA, Ruano R, Cass DL, Olutoye OO. Fetoscopic Repair of Meningomyelocele. Obstet Gynecol 2015; 126(4): 881-4.
[http://dx.doi.org/10.1097/AOG.0000000000000835] [PMID: 25923030]

[52]   Giné C, Arévalo S, Maíz N, *et al.* Fetoscopic two☐layer closure of open neural tube defects. Ultrasound Obstet Gynecol 2018; 52(4): 452-7.
[http://dx.doi.org/10.1002/uog.19104] [PMID: 29876992]

[53]   Blumenfeld YJ, Belfort MA. Updates in fetal spina bifida repair. Curr Opin Obstet Gynecol 2018; 30(2): 123-9.
[http://dx.doi.org/10.1097/GCO.0000000000000443] [PMID: 29489502]

[54]   Sanz Cortes M, Chmait RH, Lapa DA, Belfort MA, Carreras E, Miller JL, *et al.* Experience of 300 cases of prenatal fetoscopic open spina bifida repair: report of the International Fetoscopic Neural Tube Defect Repair Consortium. Am J Obstet Gynecol 2021; 225(6): e1-e11.
[http://dx.doi.org/10.1016/j.ajog.2021.05.044]

CHAPTER 5

Fetoscopy Techniques for Myelomeningocele

William Omar Contreras López[1,*], Jezid Miranda Quintero[2], Cristóbal Abello Munárriz[3], Guido Parra Anaya[4], Kai-Uwe Lewandroski[5,6,7], Juan David Hernandez[8] and **Miguel Parra Saavedra[9]**

[1] *Clínica Foscal Internacional, Autopista Floridablanca - Girón, Km 7, Floridablanca, Santander, Colombia*

[2] *Departamento de Ginecología, Facultad de medicina, Grupo de Investigación en Cuidado Intensivo y Obstetricia (GRICIO), Universidad de Cartagena, Cartagena de Indias*

[3] *Centro Médico CEDIUL, CEDIFETAL, Barranquilla, Colombia Departamento Cirugía Pediátrica y neonatal mínimamente invasiva, Universidad Metropolitana de Barranquilla, Barranquilla, Colombia*

[4] *Departamento de Ginecología y Obstetricia, División de Medicina Maternofetal, Clínica General del Norte, Barranquilla, Colombia*

[5] *Center for Advanced Spine Care of Southern Arizona and Surgical Institute of Tucson, Tucson, AZ, USA*

[6] *Departmemt of Orthopaedics, Fundación Universitaria Sanitas, Bogotá, D.C., Colombia*

[7] *Department of Neurosurgery in the Video-Endoscopic Postgraduate Program at the Universidade Federal do Estado do Rio de Janeiro - UNIRIO, Rio de Janeiro, Brazil*

[8] *Sociedad Colombiana de Anestesiología, Departamento Anestesiología, Clínica General del Norte, Barranquilla, Colombia*

[9] *Departamento de Ginecología y Obstetricia, División de Medicina Maternofetal, Clínica General del Norte, Barranquilla, Colombia*

Abstract: Myelomeningocele (MMC) repair was traditionally performed postpartum. Developmental delay, neurological deficits, and the need for shunting are persistent problems associated with this type of repair. Alternative open prenatal repairs have been proposed. Clinical studies suggest improved short-term neurological outcomes with percutaneous minimally invasive and intrauterine fetoscopic techniques using endoscopes, when compared with an open prenatal or postnatal repair. In this chapter, the authors present the various currently practiced forms of percutaneous fetoscopic MMC repair. These are frequently carried out *via* externalization of the uterus through a maternal laparotomy. The primary limitations of these procedures are preterm premature rupture of membranes (PPROM) and dehiscence or leakage at the MMC repair. The authors also present their preferred three-layer repair technique and their clinical outcomes of a small case series performed to date. Their results suggest several benefits of the full percutaneous fetoscopic technique, including a lower risk of preterm

* **Corresponding author William Omar Contreras López:** Clínica Foscal Internacional, Autopista Floridablanca - Girón, Km 7, Floridablanca, Santander, Colombia; Tel: +573112957003; E-mail: wcontreras127@unab.edu.co

labor, reduced need for postnatal revisions, and improved newborn maturity with higher gestational age. The authors conclude that fetoscopy may also offer better management of the membranes and primary closure of uterine port sites. The long-term cognitive, behavioral, and functional outcomes of fetoscopic MMC repair will need to be studied. Additional clinical outcome studies should show whether caesarean section may be required for delivery in subsequent pregnancies following the use of the fetoscopic technique to avoid uterine rupture that is commonplace after traditional open prenatal MMC repair. With the authors' technique, spontaneous vaginal delivery at term is feasible.

Keywords: Developmental delay, Intrauterine fetoscopic techniques, Myelomeningocele, Neurological deficits, Postpartum.

INTRODUCTION TO FETOSCOPY TECHNIQUES

In this chapter, the authors will describe their current fetoscopy techniques.

At present, two primary procedures are performed: 1) The pure percutaneous technique and 2) the fetoscopy technique with exposure of the uterus by laparotomy. Many leading centers are members of an international consortium - the Fetal Medicine Foundation (FMF) [1]. The first author is also a member, and his center in Barranquilla, Colombia, is accredited by FMF. It is led by Dr. Belford of Texas Children's Hospital - an internationally recognized pioneering center - and provides training based on time-tested credentialing standards; requiring neurosurgeons to be trained in endoscopy and minimally invasive spinal surgery to be accredited. In recent years, these techniques have advanced significantly and gained wider acceptance. While standard uniform treatment guidelines are lacking, several well-publicized techniques [2 - 6] do exist that the authors review as the cornerstones of their local fetal MMC repair program at the Clinica Foscal Internacional, Bucaramanga, and at the General Clinic del Norte, Barranquilla, Colombia.

Percutaneous full Endoscopic Technique

The two-layer closure with three or four ports was popularized by Dr. Denise Araújo Lapa (Pedreira) who currently coordinates the Fetal Therapy Group at Hospital Infantil Sabará and works at Albert Einstein Hospital, São Paulo, Brazil [7]. The established inclusion criteria are as follows:

- Localized neural tube defect at any level, provided the parents understand the severity of the defect and its clinical consequences,
- Gestational age at the time of surgery between 24-28.9 weeks,
- Presence of hindbrain hernia,
- No other major abnormalities, and

- A normal karyotype

Exclusion criteria include:

- Placenta previa,
- Alloimmunization,
- Multiple gestations,
- Positive HIV serology,
- Hepatitis B or C, and
- Maternal conditions that increase the risk of surgery or anesthesia such as diabetes or uncontrolled hypertension

Procedural Steps

Under general anesthesia, an ultrasound-guided amnio-infusion of 500 mL of warm saline is performed, followed by percutaneous insertion of four trocars according to the Seldinger technique using three 11 French vascular ports (Terumo, Tokyo, Japan) and one laparoscopic needle-tipped trocar employing a 5-mm balloon (Applied Medical, Rancho Santa Margarita, CA, USA). Subsequently, almost all of the amniotic fluid is removed from the uterine cavity, and a pressure-limited uterine CO_2 insufflation with a mean pressure of 14 mm Hg is performed. The typical intrauterine pressure ranges between 10 to 18 mmHg with a flow rate of 30 ml/min. Humidified CO_2 is used for the insufflation. The neurosurgical procedure involves the release of the neural placode and undermining the skin edges to allow its inline approximation. A bio-cellulose patch (Bionext, Paraná, Brazil) is placed over the defect without using sutures. In some cases, a bilateral fascial flap is raised and sutured in the midline with a 3-0 polyglycolic acid absorbable suture or with a simple continuous suture (STRATAFIXTM Spiral knotless Tissue Control Device, Ethicon, USA). If there is enough skin, it is closed over the patch with a single 2.0 monofilament, for example, a non-absorbable polypropylene stitch (Quill SRS, Angiotech, PA, USA). When skin approximation is impossible, a bilaminar skin substitute is secured (Integra Dermal Regeneration Stencil, Plainsboro, NJ, USA; or Nevelia Bi-Layer Matrix, Symatese Aesthetics, France). Two stitches are placed over the bio-cellulose patch and sutured to the skin edges using a 4-0 monofilament nylon suture. Large MMC defects can be successfully treated in utero by a full percutaneous fetoscopic technique preferring a bilaminar skin substitute over a biocellulose patch. Since February 2018, this group of authors have been using a CO_2 heating/humidification system (Insuflow, Lexion Medical, MN, USA).

Endoscopic techniques with Exteriorization of the Uterus

2-PORT TECHNIQUE WITH 3-LAYER CLOSURE [8 - 11]

Michael Belfort (Texas Children's Hospital, Houston, TX, USA)

Access procedure:

The abdomen is opened through a transverse lower abdominal incision, and the uterus is exteriorized. The fetus is gently manipulated into position with ultrasound guidance. Plication sutures (poly-4-hydroxybutyrate 2/0; Monomax, Aesculap, Center Valley, PA, USA) are placed to fix the membranes to the uterine wall before placing a 12 French port (Cook Inc., IA, USA) between the sutures and in the amniotic cavity using the Seldinger technique.

Between 300 and 500 mL of amniotic fluid is withdrawn, and the uterus is insufflated with CO_2 at 0.5 L/minute to achieve a pressure of 12 ± 2 mm Hg. A warmer/humidifier (Insuflow, Lexion Medical, MN, USA) is used. A modified FDA-approved straight endoscope allowing passage of a 5 French grasper (Karl Storz, Tuttlingen, Germany) is placed into the gas bag *via* a port. A second port is placed under vision through which 2 mm Storz scissors and a 3 mm needle holder are placed.

Neurosurgical procedure:

After placode dissection, a bovine collagen patch (Durepair, Medtronic, Goleta, CA, USA) is placed over the plate, and bilateral dura-fascial or myofascial flaps are then placed depending on the amount of muscle available, with cuts parallel to the spinal defect. These flaps are then sutured in the midline using interrupted polyglactin sutures such as vicryl (Ethicon, Somerville, NJ, USA). The skin over the flaps is then closed with interrupted poly-4-hydroxybutyrate sutures. All sutures have a straight needle to pass through the 12 French port. If necessary, skin-relaxing incisions 15 to 20 mm lateral to the defect are created to allow apposition of the skin edges in the midline. Slip knots are tied extracorporeally and placed with a knot pusher (Karl Storz, Tuttlingen, Germany).

3-PORT TECHNIQUE WITH 2/3 LAYER CLOSURE [12]

José Luis Peiro (Cincinnati Children's Hospital, Cincinnati, OH, USA),

William Omar Contreras, Miguel Parra, Guido Parra, Cristobal Abello, Juan David Hernandez; Jezid Miranda (General Clinic of the North, Barranquilla, COLOMBIA).

Access procedure:

A lower Pfannenstiel laparotomy is performed to expose the uterus. The fetus is then manipulated into position, and the best site for port insertion is determined using ultrasound to identify the placenta's location. In contrast to the established three or four stitch technique, our preferred technique is to place only two 3-0 vicryl stitches through the uterine wall to retract the uterine membranes and create a safe working space. Then, three trocars (size 12 French), using the Seldinger technique in combination with ultrasound guidance, are inserted in a triangular configuration without damaging the placenta. From then on, direct endoscopic visualization is employed, and the location of the placenta is easily identified to avoid injury to this vital structure. The trocars are secured to the uterine wall by tying the vicryl stitches through the membranes directly to the trocars. Introducing a foley catheter through the access trocar facilitates insufflation and minimizes uterine manipulation *via* the angulation of the instruments when trying to reach the pathology. Amniotic fluid is partially withdrawn to increase the working space. Heated CO_2 is insufflated at 8bmm Hg pressure at a flow rate of 3 L/min into the uterus (Fig. **1**). A 3-0 prolene stitch is employed to fix the sacral area to the uterine. This procedural step facilitates the repair of the placode by holding the fetus in a fixed position in proximity to the access portals.

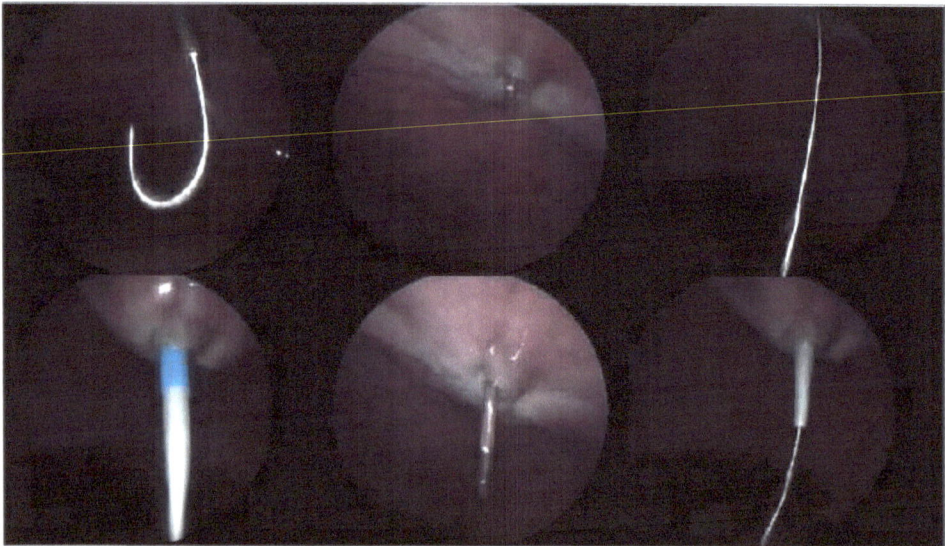

Fig. (1). The step-by-step insertion of the trocars (size 12 French) using the Seldinger technique with ultrasound guidance and direct endoscopic visualization is shown. The three ports should be placed in a triangle with a distance of 5 cm to 7 cm between them. The camera is placed in the middle port. The amniotic fluid is partially removed and replaced with heated CO_2, insufflated at pressures between 8 to 10 mm Hg into the uterus.

Neurosurgical Procedure:

The neurosurgical repair involves carefully releasing the placode and placing one or two dural substitute patches to cover the spinal defect and protect the placode. The skin defect is then closed primarily with absorbable 3-0 V-loc sutures, or if primary closure is not possible, sutured skin substitutes may be used instead. Membranes are not folded before port insertion, but port sites are always closed with absorbable sutures after removal. Tocolytics are continued, and patients are carefully monitored with serial fetal imaging and prenatal testing until delivery (Fig. **2-4**).

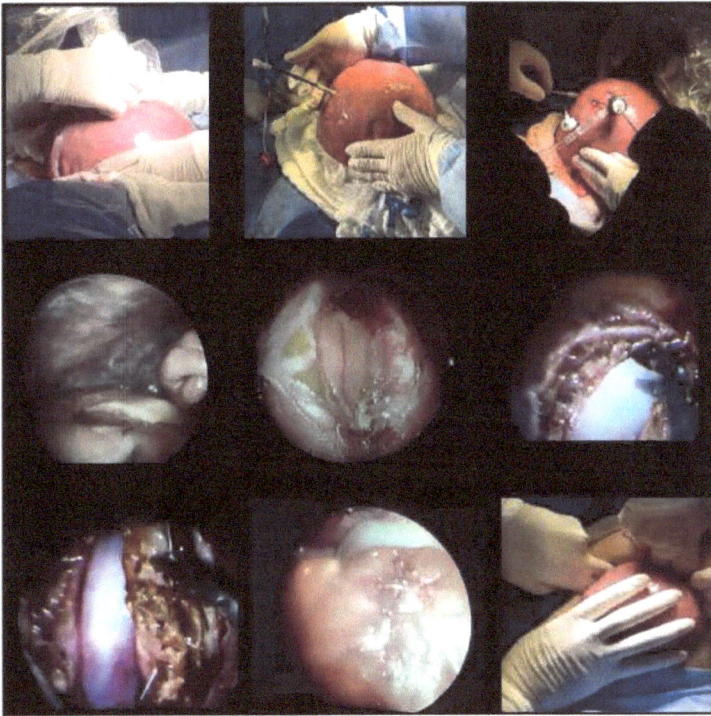

Fig. (2). Step-by-step images of the 3-port fetoscopy technique performed in Colombia by the first author are shown. The maternal-fetal team exteriorizes the uterus through a laparotomy. The fetus is then manipulated into position, and the location of the placenta is determined with ultrasound. Then, the best sites for port insertion are chosen. Three trocars, size 6, 10, and 12 Fr, are inserted using the Seldinger technique. This access procedure is conducted with ultrasound guidance and direct endoscopic visualization. Amniotic fluid is partially withdrawn, and heated CO_2 at a pressure of 8 to 10 mm Hg is used to insufflate the uterus. Subsequently, the careful release of the placode is performed, followed by the placement of one or two dural substitute patches to cover the spinal defect and protect the placode. The skin defect is then primarily closed with 3-0 V-loc absorbable sutures or 4-0 prolene sutures with interrupted stitches. The uterus is reintroduced, and tocolytics are administered. The patient is extubated and remains in the ICU for one or two days for fetal and maternal monitoring.

2-PORT TECHNIQUE WITH 1-LAYER CLOSURE [13]

Jena Miller (Johns Hopkins Center for Fetal Therapy, Baltimore, MA, USA

Access procedure:

The 2-port technique with 1-layer closure, as advocated by Miller, requires preservation of the movement of the lower extremities as an extra inclusion criterion in addition to those backed by the MOMs trial. For the exposure, a transverse lower abdominal incision is made through which exteriorization of the uterus is accomplished. The external version is performed when necessary to orient the fetus in the cephalic presentation. The location of the placenta and fetal position determine the upper port's location. Two 2-0 polyglactin sutures (Vicryl, Ethicon, Somerville, NJ, USA) are used to fold the membranes to the uterine wall, and two 12 French ports (Cook Inc., IA, USA) are placed. Amnio-reduction is followed by CO_2 insufflation at a pressure of 8 to 10 mm Hg. Warmed and humidified CO_2 (Insuflow, Lexion Medical, MN, USA) is then used for insufflation. A second port is placed in line with the defect approximately 5 cm from the initial port under direct visualization using a Lotta ventriculoscope (Karl Storz, Tuttlingen, Germany).

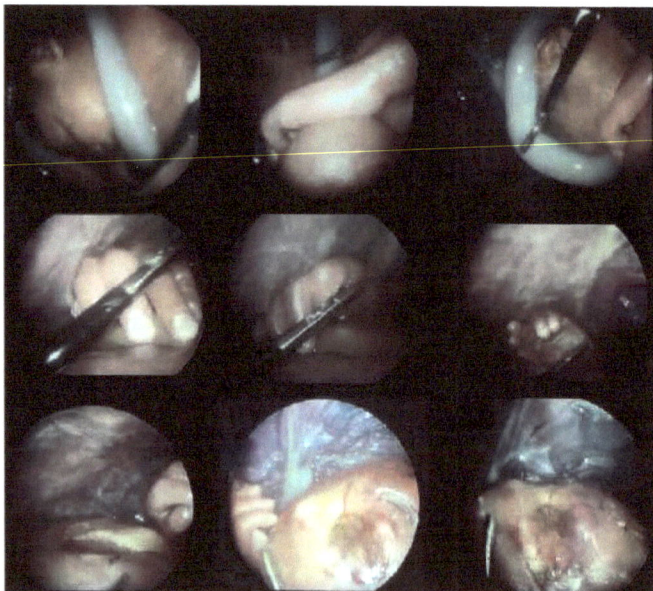

Fig. (3). Difficulties in positioning the fetus to visualize the spina bifida defect to perform a good MMC repair. In this exemplary case, the fetus presented a double circular neck, which had to be carefully withdrawn to turn the fetus to expose the spine. This maneuver was achieved by mobilizing the cord with a 2 mm diameter open grasper forceps.

Neurosurgical procedure:

The placode is released with 2 mm scissors (Karl Storz, Tuttlingen, Germany), with subsequent skin closure using interrupted 3-0 poliglecaprone sutures (Monocryl, Ethicon, Somerville, NJ, USA) and a 2 mm endoscopic needle driver (Karl Storz, Tuttlingen, Germany) in a single-layer approach. Relaxing incisions are considered if necessary to allow for primary skin closure but are rarely required. For tocolysis, indomethacin (100 mg) is given preoperatively and magnesium sulfate is started after induction of anesthesia (4 g bolus and then 2 g/hr). Postoperatively, indomethacin is continued at a maximum dose of 50 mg every 6 hours for 48 hours, but is generally tapered off as soon as possible. Nifedipine 1020 mg every 6 - 8 hours is started if there is concern about uterine irritability or premature contractions. Vaginal progesterone (200 mg) is also continued every night after surgery. Cervical cup pessary (Bioteque, San José, CA, USA) is offered for cervical shortening < 25 mm.

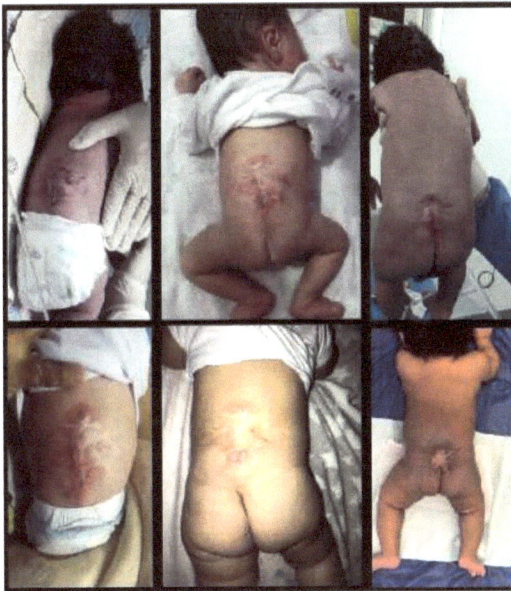

Fig. (4). . Several cases of intrauterine fetoscopy MMC repairs healed at birth are shown (top panel). The bottom panel shows the healed MMC defect at two months postpartum. The pictured repairs were carried out at the General Clinic del Norte, Barranquilla, Colombia.

Case Examples

To date, 8 cases of intrauterine fetoscopic MMC repair with a mean gestational age of 34.5 weeks, but no less than 31 weeks, have been performed at the General Clinic del Norte, Barranquilla, Colombia. Premature rupture of membranes (PPROM) and preterm labor remain challenging, but CO_2 heating/humidification appears to decrease their occurrence and increase gestational age at birth. Long-term follow-up analysis of clinical outcomes is ongoing.

Case 1

An ultrasound and magnetic resonance image diagnosed a lumbosacral MMC of L3-L5 in a 24-year-old primiparous mother with a 26-week pregnancy. The male fetus had hydrocephalus and Chiari II malformation with decreased cerebellar tonsils. The karyotype was negative for other abnormalities. With prior approval from the patient and her family and the institution's ethics committee, the fetoscopy was performed using the 3-port, 2-layer technique. Under maternal general anesthesia, a transverse Giordano-Cherney-type incision was made, and the uterus was exteriorized. Then, three 10-Fr cannulas were introduced between the uterine wall and the amniotic cavity. The membranes were fixed with two parallel PDS points using 2-0 sutures. The amniotic fluid was extracted, and humidified warm CO_2 was insufflated. The fetus received intramuscular anesthesia consisting of rocuronium, fentanyl, and atropine). The fetus's cardiovascular function was monitored with real-time ultrasound. Constant uterine humidification was employed. The initial coagulation of the membrane was performed with an electric scalpel, followed by dissection of the placode with microscissors, carefully freeing the neural tissue from surrounding tissues. A dural patch (Duragen-Integra®) was then placed over the defect. A 3 mm straight trocar was employed for the medullary retubulization, and was secured with individual stitches. Myofascial flaps were cut parallel to the spinal defect, which was then sutured in the midline with monocryl 4-0. Subcutaneous skin dissection was performed by suturing it with end-knots of prolene 3-0, thus achieving a triple-layer closure. The instruments were removed, and the trocar insertion sites were closed with 2-0 chromic catgut. The total surgical time was 4 hours and 20 minutes, of which the dissection and repair time was 2 hours, achieving tight closure of the defect without intraoperative complications.

The gestational age at the time of surgery was 26.3 weeks, and the duration of surgery (skin-to-skin time) was 254 minutes, of which 102 minutes was fetoscopic surgery. No maternal complications occurred. The baby was born by caesarean section due to the detection of labor with a gestational age of 37.3 weeks and a birth weight of 2,910 grams. At birth, the skin defect was already adequately healed. The newborn vigorously mobilized his legs, and at the 18-month follow-up, he no longer presented with Arnold Chiari malformation, and there was no evidence of hydrocephalus. To date, he has not required a ventriculoperitoneal shunt, nor does he have a cerebrospinal fluid leak through the MMC repair (Fig. **5**).

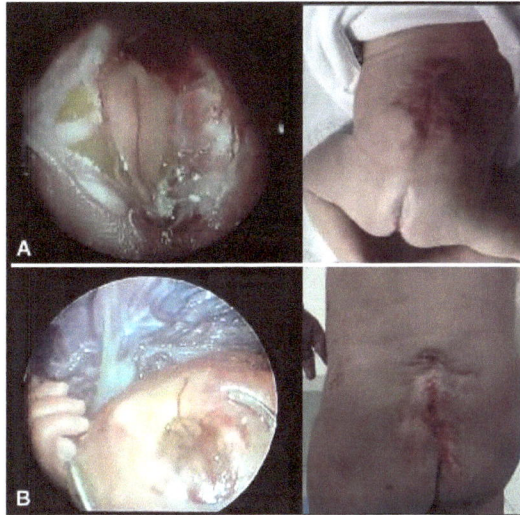

Fig. (5). Image A, case 1: Fetoscopic intraoperative view of the L3-L5 defect is shown on the left. On the right, the location of the lesion at birth is pictured. The baby was delivered by cesarean section due to the detection of labor with a gestational age of 37.3 weeks and a birth weight of 2,910 grams without a CSF fistula. There was no need for DVP at the 18-month follow-up. Image B, Case 2: Fetoscopic visualization of intraoperative left L4-sacrum MMC fetoscopic lesion repair. The patient was born vaginally at 39.2 weeks of gestation, without a CSF fistula, with adequate mobilization of the legs, and without the need for DVP at the 12-month follow-up. The pictured repairs were performed at the General Clinic del Norte, Barranquilla, Colombia.

Case 2

This case involved a fetus from a multi-pregnancy mother, presenting a myeloschisis lesion from L4 to the sacrum with herniation of the rhombencephalon and moderate ventriculomegaly (10/13 mm). Surgery was performed at 26 weeks. Relaxing incisions were required to close the lesion in two layers with skin closure over a patch. The baby was born at 39 weeks gestation and *via* vaginal delivery. At birth, there was evidence of reversal of the hindbrain herniation (C2) without hydrocephalus, with adequate healing of the defect, without CSF fistula, and with preserved motor function. To our knowledge, this was the first fetus born in Latin America by vaginal delivery at term following fetoscopy with the 3-port technique; being delivered at 39 weeks and weighing 3,800 grams. The incisions in the uterus were so small that the mother was able to enter labor, becoming a milestone in the development of fetal medicine and surgery in the country. The case established a new standard in the management of this pathology in Colombia; reducing its impact on fetuses and their families, and providing the benefits of intrauterine repair while minimizing the risks for the baby and mother with a minimally invasive technique.

Case 3

This female fetus was also from a multi-pregnancy mother, presenting myelomeningocele from L2 to L5 with herniation of the rhombencephalon and moderate ventriculomegaly (10/13 mm). The fetus moved her legs during sonography, and no other malformations were noted; therefore, fetoscopic repair of the defect was indicated. The procedure was performed at 26 weeks gestation using the three-port technique. The baby was born *via* C-section at 38 weeks and was mature, did not need any support measures to thrive and was returned to her mother immediately after birth. The initial screening examination after birth showed spontaneous movements in the lower extremities, feet including toes without foot deformity, and normal natal reflexes indicating normal neurological function. A postpartum MRI of the head and neck area showed that the previously diagnosed Arnold-Chiari Malformation had resolved (Fig. **6**).

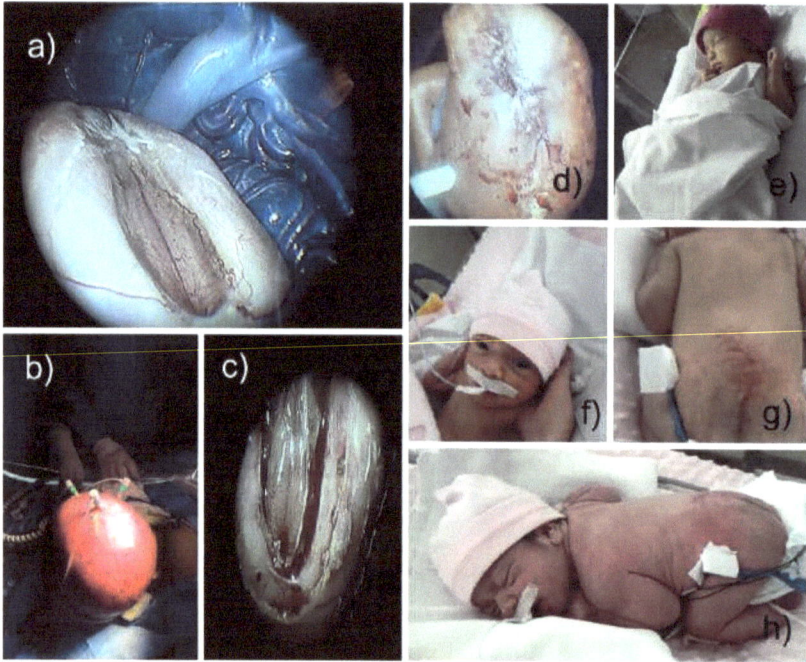

Fig. (6). Case 3: a) Fetoscopic intraoperative view of the L2-L5 defect is shown at 26 weeks of gestation. b) Uterus exposed through a low Pfannenstiel incision. No incision was made in the uterus. Three 12-French portals were placed using the Seldinger technique. c) Intrauterine endoscopic view of the significant raphe defect. Two longitudinal incisions were made on each side of the placode into the thin dysplastic epithelium to facilitate closure with interrupted stitches, as shown in image (d). e) The baby was delivered by caesarean section as a mature newborn at 38 weeks gestation with a birth weight of 2,800 grams, without a CSF fistula, and with a 35 cm head circumference. C-section was chosen because the mother had two previous C-section deliveries. In the absence of contraindication, a vaginal delivery is possible.

DISCUSSION

The main limitations of percutaneous fetoscopic MMC repair are premature rupture of membranes (PPROM) and dehiscence or leakage at the MMC repair site that require postnatal revision [14 - 16]. This percutaneous fetoscopic approach to MMC repair may offer a better alternative to the open approach if the technique can be optimized to overcome preterm labor, PPROM, and the need for postnatal revision surgeries of the repair. Gestational age at birth should further improve with better management of the membranes and primary closure of uterine port sites. This advantage is seen when fetoscopic MMC repair is achieved by maternal laparotomy. The long-term cognitive, behavioral, and functional outcomes of fetoscopic MMC repair have yet to be determined and compared to the gold standard of open fetal MMC repair. After open fetal surgery, a caesarean section is required for delivery in subsequent pregnancies because of the possibility of uterine rupture. According to the recently published results on more than 300 cases of repair by fetoscopy with externalization of the uterus [17], the fetoscopic repair of MMC by maternal laparotomy, proposed by Belfort *et al.* [8 - 10], has clear advantages. This technique used in our center often allows vaginal, spontaneous term delivery, as we have reported in our cases.

CONCLUSION

The development of formal clinical guidelines for fetoscopic MMC repair is on the agenda of the few centers worldwide that perform these risky and technically challenging procedures on unborn fetuses. The authors are advocates of prenatal repair with minimally invasive and endoscopic techniques, considering this to be a way to further reduce the risk of MMC repairs and improve neurological function and the affected individuals' quality of life.

REFERENCES

[1]   Sanz Cortes M, Lapa DA, Acacio GL, *et al.* Proceedings of the First Annual Meeting of the International Fetoscopic Myelomeningocele Repair Consortium. Ultrasound Obstet Gynecol 2019; 53(6): 855-63.
[http://dx.doi.org/10.1002/uog.20308] [PMID: 31169957]

[2]   Corroenne R, Yepez M, Pyarali M, *et al.* Longitudinal evaluation of motor function in patients who underwent prenatal or postnatal neural tube defect repair. Ultrasound Obstet Gynecol 2021; 58(2): 221-9.
[http://dx.doi.org/10.1002/uog.22165] [PMID: 32730648]

[3]   Corroenne R, Yepez M, Pyarali M, *et al.* Prenatal predictors of motor function in children with open spina bifida: a retrospective cohort study. BJOG 2021; 128(2): 384-91.
[http://dx.doi.org/10.1111/1471-0528.16538] [PMID: 32975898]

[4]   Corroenne R, Zhu KH, Johnson E, *et al.* Impact of the size of the lesion in prenatal neural tube defect repair on imaging, neurosurgical and motor outcomes: a retrospective cohort study. BJOG 2021; 128(2): 392-9.
[http://dx.doi.org/10.1111/1471-0528.16316] [PMID: 32406575]

[5]   Cruz-Martínez R, Chavelas-Ochoa F, Martínez-Rodríguez M, *et al.* Open Fetal Microneurosurgery for Intrauterine Spina Bifida Repair. Fetal Diagn Ther 2021; 48(3): 163-73.
        [http://dx.doi.org/10.1159/000513311] [PMID: 33582666]

[6]   Protzenko T, Bellas A, Pousa MS, *et al.* Reviewing the prognostic factors in myelomeningocele. Neurosurg Focus 2019; 47(4)E2
        [http://dx.doi.org/10.3171/2019.7.FOCUS19462] [PMID: 31574474]

[7]   Lapa DA. Endoscopic fetal surgery for neural tube defects. Best Pract Res Clin Obstet Gynaecol 2019; 58: 133-41.
        [http://dx.doi.org/10.1016/j.bpobgyn.2019.05.001] [PMID: 31350160]

[8]   Belfort MA, Whitehead WE, Shamshirsaz AA, *et al.* Fetoscopic Open Neural Tube Defect Repair. Obstet Gynecol 2017; 129(4): 734-43.
        [http://dx.doi.org/10.1097/AOG.0000000000001941] [PMID: 28277363]

[9]   Belfort MA, Whitehead WE, Shamshirsaz AA, *et al.* Comparison of two fetoscopic open neural tube defect repair techniques: single□ *vs* three□layer closure. Ultrasound Obstet Gynecol 2020; 56(4): 532-40.
        [http://dx.doi.org/10.1002/uog.21915] [PMID: 31709658]

[10]   Belfort MA, Whitehead WE, Shamshirsaz AA, Ruano R, Cass DL, Olutoye OO. Fetoscopic Repair of Meningomyelocele. Obstet Gynecol 2015; 126(4): 881-4.
        [http://dx.doi.org/10.1097/AOG.0000000000000835] [PMID: 25923030]

[11]   Blumenfeld YJ, Belfort MA. Updates in fetal spina bifida repair. Curr Opin Obstet Gynecol 2018; 30(2): 123-9.
        [http://dx.doi.org/10.1097/GCO.0000000000000443] [PMID: 29489502]

[12]   Patel SK, Habli MA, McKinney DN, *et al.* Fetoscopic Multilayer, Dural Patch Closure Technique for Intrauterine Myelomeningocele Repair: 2-Dimensional Operative Video. Oper Neurosurg (Hagerstown) 2021; 20(2): E131-2.
        [http://dx.doi.org/10.1093/ons/opaa309] [PMID: 33047136]

[13]   Miller JL, Groves ML, Ahn ES, *et al.* Implementation Process and Evolution of a Laparotomy-Assisted 2-Port Fetoscopic Spina Bifida Closure Program. Fetal Diagn Ther 2021; 48(8): 603-10.
        [http://dx.doi.org/10.1159/000518507] [PMID: 34518445]

[14]   Adzick NS. Fetal surgery for myelomeningocele: trials and tribulations. J Pediatr Surg 2012; 47(2): 273-81.
        [http://dx.doi.org/10.1016/j.jpedsurg.2011.11.021] [PMID: 22325376]

[15]   Johnson MP, Bennett KA, Rand L, Burrows PK, Thom EA, Howell LJ, *et al.* The Management of Myelomeningocele Study: obstetrical outcomes and risk factors for obstetrical complications following prenatal surgery. Am J Obstet Gynecol 2016; 215(6): e1-9.
        [http://dx.doi.org/10.1016/j.ajog.2016.07.052]

[16]   Lapa Pedreira DA, Acacio GL, Gonçalves RT, *et al.* Percutaneous fetoscopic closure of large open spina bifida using a bilaminar skin substitute. Ultrasound Obstet Gynecol 2018; 52(4): 458-66.
        [http://dx.doi.org/10.1002/uog.19001] [PMID: 29314321]

[17]   Sanz Cortes M, Chmait RH, Lapa DA, Belfort MA, Carreras E, Miller JL, *et al.* Experience of 300 cases of prenatal fetoscopic open spina bifida repair: report of the International Fetoscopic Neural Tube Defect Repair Consortium. Am J Obstet Gynecol 2021; 225(6): e1-e11.
        [http://dx.doi.org/10.1016/j.ajog.2021.05.044]

CHAPTER 6

Microendoscopic Intradural Cordotomy for the Treatment of Cancer Pain

William Omar Contreras López[1,*], Erich Talamoni Fonoff[2], Kai-Uwe Lewandrowski[3,4,5] and Jorge Felipe Ramírez León[6,7,8]

[1] *Clínica Foscal Internacional, Autopista Floridablanca - Girón, Km 7, Floridablanca, Santander, Colombia*

[2] *Division of Functional Neurosurgery of Institute of Psychiatry, Department of Neurology, University of São Paulo Medical School, São Paulo, Brazil*

[3] *Center for Advanced Spine Care of Southern Arizona and Surgical Institute of Tucson, Tucson, AZ, USA*

[4] *Departmemt of Orthopaedics, Fundación Universitaria Sanitas, Bogotá, D.C., Colombia*

[5] *Department of Neurosurgery in the Video-Endoscopic Postgraduate Program at the Universidade Federal do Estado do Rio de Janeiro - UNIRIO, Rio de Janeiro, Brazil*

[6] *Minimally Invasive Spine Center. Bogotá, D.C., Colombia*

[7] *Reina Sofía Clinic. Bogotá, D.C., Colombia*

[8] *Fundación Universitaria Sanitas. Bogotá, D.C., Colombia*

Abstract: Spinal chordotomy is an alternative to analgesic opioid therapy, nerve blocks, and subcutaneous or intravenous techniques for cancer-induced pain. Patients with advanced metastatic disease require significant pain relief. Unfortunately, not all patients respond well to the standard therapies. For these patients, cordotomy offers a potential breakthrough. Cordotomy involves thermally disrupting the nociceptive pathways in the anterior spinothalamic tract to interrupt pain transmission from the spinal cord to the brain. The anterior spinothalamic tract is responsible for somatic pain sensations, touch, and temperature discrimination. This chapter presents an endoscopic-assisted percutaneous anterolateral radiofrequency intradural cordotomy technique. The entire procedure is done under direct endoscopic visualization of the cervical spinal cord. The authors provide an up-to-date summary of targeted minimally invasive pain intervention, which utilizes controlled electrical stimulation to confirm the physiological target. It is associated with less trauma to surrounding spinal tissue and lower risks due to vascular injury or adverse effects of intrathecal contrast.

* **Corresponding author William Omar Contreras López:** NEMOD International Neuromodulation Center; Clínica Foscal Internacional Floridablanca, Hospital Internacional de Colombia (HIC); Tel: +573112957003; E-mail: wcontreras127@unab.edu.co

Keywords: Analgesic opioid therapy, Cordotomy, Metastatic disease, Nerve blocks, Spinal chordotomy.

INTRODUCTION

Cancer can elicit pain by invading or destroying neighboring tissues. Additionally, tumor growth may exert pressure on nerves, bones, or organs, leading to pain. Another contributing factor is the release of pain-inducing chemicals by the tumor. Such pain can be managed through non-invasive methods, including analgesics and optimized opioid therapy, and semi-invasive approaches, such as nerve blocks and subcutaneous, intravenous, or spinal infusion techniques [1]. However, not all patients experience satisfactory pain relief using these methods [2, 3]. For these individuals, Cordotomy represents a potentially transformative intervention. Cordotomy involves the selective disruption of nociceptive pathways in the anterior spinothalamic tract within the spinal cord, achieved through thermal techniques. This disruption effectively interrupts the transmission of pain signals.

The anterior spinothalamic tract plays a crucial role in transmitting somatic pain sensations, and facilitating touch and temperature discrimination. This study introduces an innovative technique called endoscopic-assisted percutaneous anterolateral radiofrequency cordotomy. With this approach, we aim to attain intradural endoscopic visualization of the cervical spinal cord through a percutaneous method. This allows for more precise targeting of the spinal region for anterolateral cordotomy. Importantly, this technique helps minimize the risk of unintended damage to spinal tissue or blood vessels, ensuring a safer and more accurate procedure.

Cordotomy Rationale

The quintessential insertion point for the electrode within the spinal cord is strategically located at the median juncture between the dentate ligament and the ventral root ingress zone. Leveraging endoscopic guidance obviates the excessive dependency on fluoroscopy, eliminating the necessity for intrathecal contrast deployment. Upon meticulous optimization of the neurophysiological target, a conventional radiofrequency methodology is employed for cordotomy. This modality efficaciously provides superior analgesia devoid of supplemental complications or cerebrospinal fluid extravasation. Preliminary forays utilizing this technique suggest that percutaneous endoscopic interventions offer considerable promise for precise spinal cord manipulation, thereby improving both procedural safety and efficacy. While the debate surrounding the one-needle versus two-needle technique persists, our group prefers the dual-needle modality, considering it the safer alternative (Fig. **1**).

The protocol is initiated with a lateral foray into the spinal canal at the C1-2 interstice, under the vigilant guidance of fluoroscopy. Post the successful breach into the cerebrospinal fluid (CSF) employing a guiding cannula (17-gauge needle), the endoscope is deployed, providing excellent visualization of the spinal cord and its contiguous architectures. Such endoscopic clarity proffers a highly detailed delineation of critical anatomical waypoints, inclusive of the spinal cord's pial surface, arachnoid membrane, dentate ligament, dorsal and ventral root ingress zones, and vasculature (Fig. **2**).

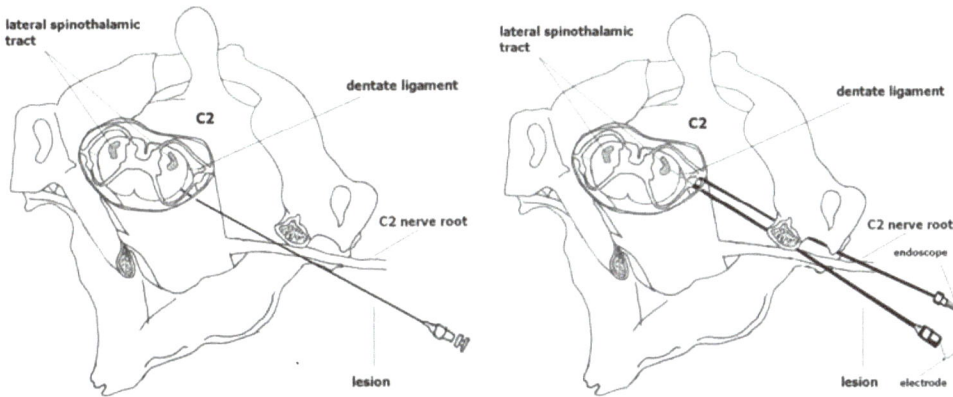

Fig. (1). Pictured; the (left) one puncture versus (right) two puncture techniques. The two ports technique allows for direct visualization of the RF electrode tip between the dentate ligament and the anterior spinal roots.

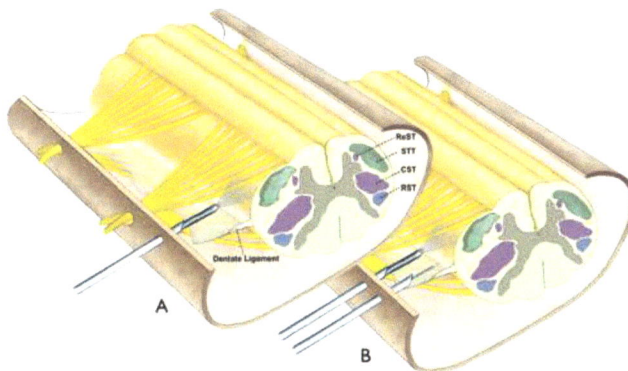

Fig. (2). Stepwise procedure for the microendoscopic cordotomy technique. Step 1: Insert the 17-gauge cannula perpendicular to the skin toward the spinal canal at the C1–2 interspace under fluoroscopic visualization. Step 2: Once the subarachnoid space is reached, the endoscope is introduced (A). Step 3: The second cannula is introduced in a parallel channel, also reaching the CSF space close to the first dural puncture (B). Step 4: Target identification followed by spinal cord puncture. Step 5: Stimulation and thermal RF lesion application, followed by intraoperative neurological examination (pinprick). CST = corticothalamic tract; ReST = reticulospinal tract; RST = rubrospinal tract. Copyright Erich Talamoni Fonoff. Published with permission. Figure is available in color online only. Neurosurg. 2016 Feb;124(2):389-96.

Exemplary Case

A 64-year-old male presented with progressive right-sided chest pain persisting for nine months, attributed to advanced lung cancer. Over time, the pain worsened and became constant, pulsatile, and highly intense (measured at 95/100mm on the visual analog scale (VAS). Despite medication usage, the pain remained resistant. It was localized to the right thorax, explicitly affecting the T3 to T7 dermatomes, likely resulting from neoplastic infiltration of the parietal pleura and chest wall. Unable to control the pain using opioids and adjuvant analgesics, the oncology clinic referred the patient for additional palliative interventions. Before the procedure, the patient provided informed consent, and the institutional ethics committee approved. Our institution follows a strict protocol for recommending ablative procedures to manage pain. Such procedures are reserved for patients with advanced cancer who have exhausted curative treatment options and continue to experience uncontrolled pain, even with opioid infusion pumps.

Step-by-step Technique

With the patient in a supine orientation and under minimal sedation, the cranium was meticulously stabilized utilizing Rosomoff's cranial fixation apparatus. Fluoroscopic guidance was judiciously employed to facilitate the precise delivery of local anesthetics to both the epidermal layer and the profound musculature of the superior lateral cervical region, a locus approximately 1 cm caudal and posterior to the mastoid prominence. Concurrently, leveraging the precision of fluoroscopy, a 17-gauge cannula was introduced orthogonally to the epidermis, oriented toward the spinal conduit at the C1-C2 interspace (refer to Fig. **3**). Upon achieving ingress to the cerebrospinal fluid (CSF) reservoir, further fluoroscopic intervention was deemed unnecessary.

Once the cannula is passed through the dura, its position becomes anchored due to the enveloping epidermis, cervical musculature, and dura; restricting its motility to mere millimeters. An endoscopic apparatus with a 0.9mm diameter (sourced from MYELOTEC, Inc., Roswell, USA), was then introduced *via* the aforementioned cannula to directly appraise the spinal conduit. This modern endoscopic mechanism provides a 70° observational scope and amplifies imagery to 40X at a 0° observational trajectory, ensuring clear visualization amidst the cerebrospinal fluid (CSF). This endoscopic view facilitates the pinpoint identification of key anatomical entities, including the pial interface of the spinal cord (SC), concomitant vasculature, the arachnoid stratum, and the dentate ligament, as well as the dorsal and ventral root ingress sectors and their affiliated radicular vasculature.

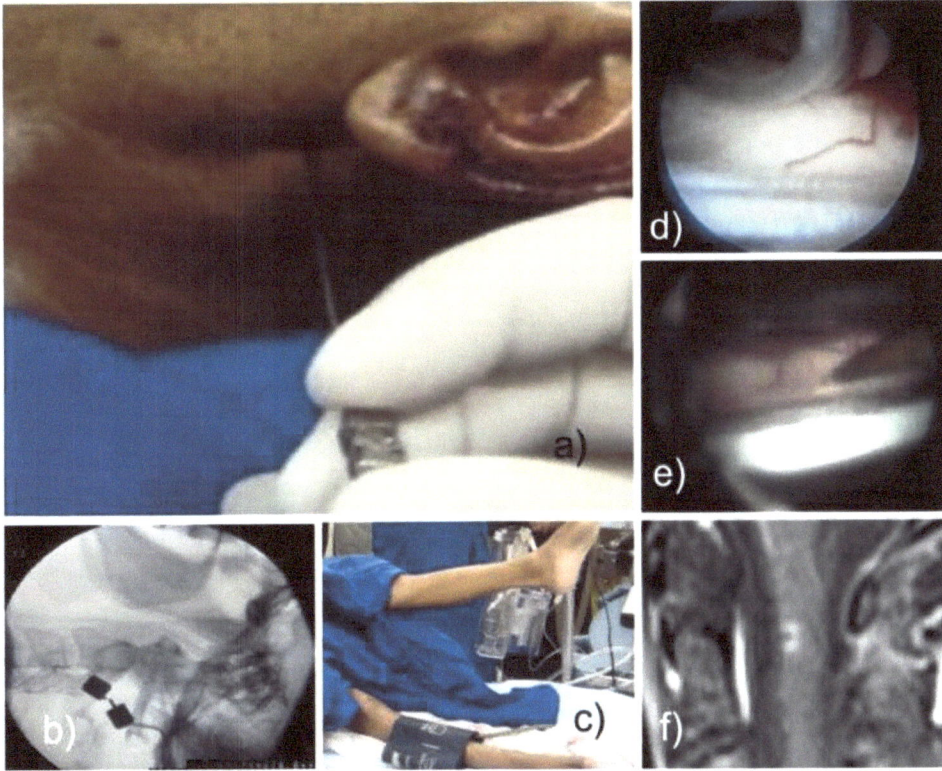

Fig. (3). A Methodical Elucidation Cordotomy: Step 1 (a,b): Employing a 17-gauge needle, a percutaneous insertion is performed orthogonally to the epidermal surface, directed towards the spinal conduit, approximately 1 cm caudal to the mastoid apex at the C1–2 interspace under the guidance of fluoroscopy. Upon attaining the subarachnoid domain, a slender endoscope (measuring 0.9mm in diameter) is seamlessly introduced *via* the needle's lumen. This maneuver facilitates the clear discernment of the dentate ligament juxtaposed with the oscillatory spinal cord.

Step 2: Subsequently, a secondary cannula is positioned on a parallel trajectory, also culminating within the CSF reservoir proximate to the first dural penetration. This conduit serves as the portal for the radiofrequency (RF) electrode, whose insertion is carefully overseen using the optic fiber (b).

Step 3: With precision, the RF electrode penetrates the lateral quadrant of the spinal cord, nestling between the dentate ligament and the anterolateral sulcus of the cord, a region delineated by the nascent spinal rootlets.

Step 4: A synthesis of electrostimulation mapping and intraoperative neurological assessment, notably pinprick testing, rigorously determines the exact spinal target. The patient's feedback regarding stimulus sensation, localized contralaterally to the puncture locus and emanating from the pain-afflicted region, becomes paramount. Stimulation currents oscillate between frequencies of 2 Hz and 50 Hz. Specifically, a 2 Hz stimulation typically elicits contractions within the longus colli musculature at a range of 0.5–1 V. Any extraneous contractions indicate that the electrode's tip is located within the corticospinal (motor) tract—a precarious position as a lesion here could precipitate muscular paresis. Such an eventuality mandates an anterior repositioning of the needle. The sensory pathways, conversely, are demarcated *via* 50 Hz stimulation. Electrode placement within the spinothalamic tract yields sensations of temperature modulations (either warmth or cold) within the corresponding contralateral bodily hemisphere at intensities ranging from 0.1–0.3 V. The intricate topographical layout of the spinothalamic tract undergoes careful evaluation during this phase, elucidating the mediolateral orientation typical of the upper and lower body representation. Upon achieving the optimal target, we proceed to a focalized thermal obliteration of the tract (as depicted in Figure c) utilizing radiofrequency with tip temperatures oscillating between 70 - 90°C sustained for 60 seconds (e). The post-operative sagittal tomography, as illustrated in Figure (f), evidences the ablative lesion, manifesting as a hyperdense signal at the craniocervical juncture.

The preferred locus for the electrode's insertion within the spinal cord emerged as an equidistant point straddling the dentate ligament and the ventral root ingress zone (refer to Fig. **3**). Post-determination of this target, the surgeon meticulously anchored the cannula, paving the way for a judicious retraction of the endoscope. This maneuver necessitated finesse, striving to retain the spinal cord's relative position to the cannula. *via* the endoscopic view, the cannula was cautiously positioned to engage the pial exterior precisely over the target.

Leveraging the same conduit, the radiofrequency electrode engages the pial veneer of the spinal cord at the selected locus. The movement of the electrode within the spinal domain is steered by traditional impedance readings—CSF oscillating around an impedance of 200Ω, juxtaposed against the spinal cord's substantial measure of approximately 800Ω.

Subsequently, a regimented electrical stimulation, operating at a frequency spectrum of 5075 Hz coupled with a 1 ms pulse width, is conducted. This aims to corroborate the precision of the target, invoking a distinct tingling sensation in the contralateral thoracic expanse, encompassing the pain-affected territory. This feedback is undertaken with the patient's conscious involvement, rendering them integral to the procedure. The ablation process employs radiofrequency, elevating the thermal gradient to 75°C sustained over a minute. In this illustrative scenario, a pair of consecutive ablations procured the desired thermoanalgesic effect on the body's contralateral facet, reaching spinal elevations proximal to the clavicular demarcation.

Post-ablation, the endoscope was re-engaged within the cerebrospinal fluid (CSF) milieu, illuminating the region of the pial overlay of the spinal cord where the electrode had previously been positioned. Utilizing the aforementioned cannula, the radiofrequency electrode was carefully guided to engage with the pial stratum at the pre-established locus. Throughout this perilous procedure, neither haemorrhagic episodes nor other complications arose. Furthermore, the postoperative follow-up remained devoid of any CSF exudation, either immediately following the operation or during the protracted recovery phase. Concomitant with the palpable analgesic relief, some patients might manifest an ipsilateral Horner's manifestation and nuanced upper extremity ataxia—typical transient effects associated with percutaneous radiofrequency cordotomies. In the paradigmatic case at hand, the ataxia spanned a period of nine days, eventually waning after the two-week mark. At the half-year postoperative evaluation, the patient exhibited sustained pain relief, quantified by a visual analog scale (VAS) at an impressive 0/100mm. The electrode's movements within the spinal sanctum were guided by traditional impedance metrics, with the CSF and spinal cord registering approximations of 200Ω and 800Ω, respectively. A calibrated electrical signal, set at a frequency of 50Hz and a pulse width of 1 ms, was used to validate the electrode's precise location, evidenced by eliciting a specific contralateral thoracic tingling sensation encompassing the pain-afflicted domain. Such precise feedback relies on the patient's lucid cognizance and active procedural involvement. The thermal ablation modus operandi employed radiofrequency elevation, achieving 75°C sustained for a minute's duration. In this distinct exemplar, a pair of sequential ablations were used to achieve the desired thermoanalgesic effect, radiating contralaterally to spinal altitudes in proximity to the clavicular boundary.

Endoscopic Equipment

We used Mylotec® endoscopes, which are available in 3 resolutions ranging from 3000E to 3030E, with a higher pixel count resulting in higher resolution pictures from 3000E (10,000-pixel fiber bundle), 3010E (15,000-pixel fiber bundle), and 3030E (30,000-pixel fiber bundle). An array of eyepiece couplers may be used, with lens sizes ranging from 25mm to 32mm and 40mm. The size of the lens, the eyepiece coupler, and the video system ultimately determine the image size on the video monitor. Endoscopic systems are available with a 70-degree field of view or a zero angle. The focal range is approximately 5mm to 20mm. Light from a light source is carried through a light cable to the light input connecter of the scope. Light is carried to the end of the endoscope in the larger fibers which encircle the inner fiber bundle. The CCD video camera from the video tower is connected to the eyepiece coupler. The eyepiece of the endoscope connects to a standard eyepiece coupler that is a part of almost any video tower system. The components of the endoscopic system used in our cordotomy procedures are shown in Fig. (**4**).

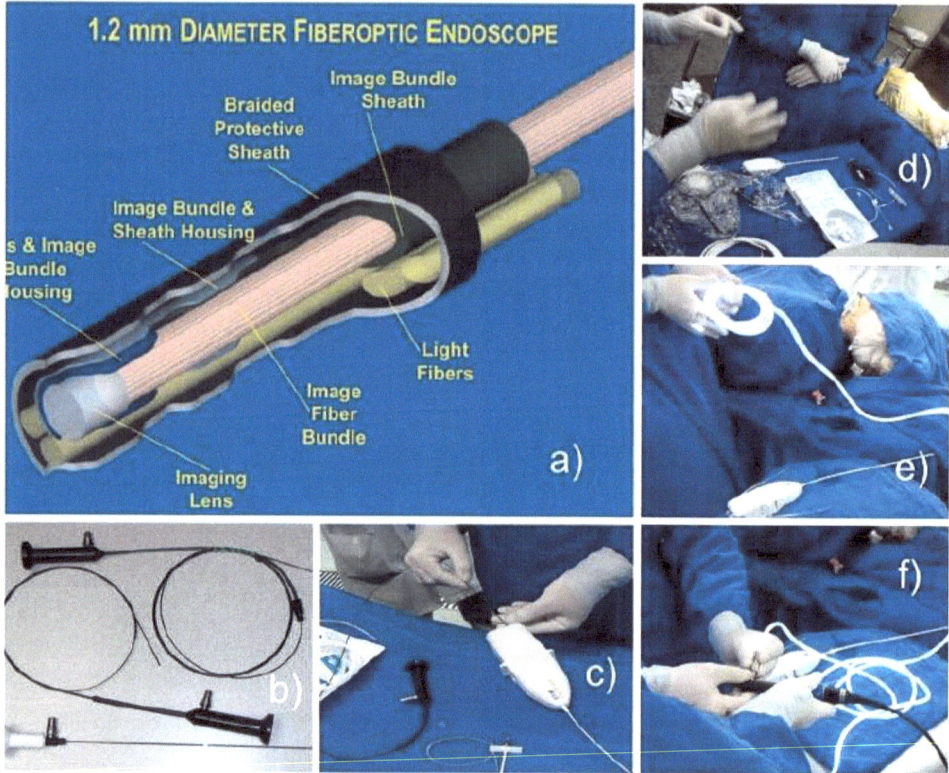

Fig. (4). The fiber optic must have a diameter able to pass through a 17-gauge needle cannula; the light is connected to the light source. A 0.9mm/1.2mm-thick endoscope (MYELOTEC, Inc., Roswell, USA) is inserted through the same cannula for a direct view of the spinal canal. This device renders a 70° field of view with a 40X image magnification at a 0° angle of view, which provides a clear image through CSF. The equipment is sterilized for every procedure.

Case-series

A cohort of twenty-four patients, composed of 62% males and 38% females, underwent the intricate endoscopic cordotomy intervention. Universal achievement of optimal pain amelioration was noted. Predominantly, pain etiologies were attributed to metastatic manifestations, evident in 38% of the subjects. Subsequent primary malignancies such as pulmonary and prostatic carcinomas accounted for 21% of the presentations. Further breakdown revealed mammary carcinoma affecting 12% of the sample, with squamous cell neoplasms being the causative factor in a subset of 8% (Refer to Table **1**).

Table 1. Clinical cordotomy series, surgical access, intraoperative findings, and outcomes.

Patient	Age	Procedure	Etiology	Surgical Access	Intraoperative Observation	Outcome
1M	55	THERAPEUTIC (Endoscopic Cordotomy)	Intractable oncologic chest pain in the right side. Lung carcinoma	Percutaneous endoscopic cordotomy C1-C2 with 17G needle in the left side	Clear endoscopic visualization of spinal cord and dentate ligament	Satisfactory control of pain
2M	56	THERAPEUTIC (Endoscopic Cordotomy)	Intractable oncologic chest pain in the left side. Lung carcinoma	Percutaneous endoscopic cordotomy C1-C2 with 17G needle in the right side	Viewed spinal cord, dentate ligament, spinal roots. Cordotomy was performed with the improvement of pain	Satisfactory control of pain
-	58	THERAPEUTIC (Endoscopic Cordotomy)	Oncologic right chest pain due to lung carcinoma	Percutaneous endoscopic cordotomy C1-C2 with 17G needle in the left side	Clear endoscopic visualization of spinal cord and dentate ligament	Satisfactory control of pain
-	63	THERAPEUTIC (Endoscopic Cordotomy)	Oncologic pain in the right arm due to breast cancer	Percutaneous endoscopic cordotomy C1-C2 with 17G needle in the left side	Clear endoscopic visualization of spinal cord and dentate ligament	Satisfactory control of pain
5M	52	THERAPEUTIC (Endoscopic Cordotomy)	Oncologic pain in right pelvis and leg due to prostate carcinoma	Percutaneous endoscopic cordotomy C1-C2 with 17G needle in the left side	Clear endoscopic visualization of spinal cord and dentate ligament	Satisfactory control of pain
6M	47	THERAPEUTIC (Endoscopic Cordotomy)	Oncologic pain in left lower limb. Carcinoma of the prostate	Percutaneous endoscopic cordotomy C1-C2 with 17G needle in the right side	Viewed spinal cord, dentate ligament, spinal roots.	Satisfactory control of pain
7M	67	THERAPEUTIC (Endoscopic Cordotomy)	Oncologic pain in the pelvis and left leg. Carcinoma de prostate	Percutaneous endoscopic cordotomy C1-C2 with 17G needle in the right side	Endoscopic visualization clear spinal cord and dentate ligament	Satisfactory control of pain

(Table 1) cont.....

Patient	Age	Procedure	Etiology	Surgical Access	Intraoperative Observation	Outcome
8M	59	THERAPEUTIC (Endoscopic Cordotomy)	Oncologic left body pain due to carcinomatosis	Percutaneous endoscopic cordotomy C1-C2 with 17G needle in the right side	Clear endoscopic visualization of spinal cord and dentate ligament	Satisfactory control of pain
-	43	THERAPEUTIC (Endoscopic Cordotomy)	Oncologic pain in left upper limb. Multiple squamous cell carcinoma	Percutaneous endoscopic cordotomy C1-C2 with 17G needle in the right side	Viewed spinal cord, dentate ligament, spinal roots. Cordotomy was peformed with improvement of pain	Satisfactory control of pain, ataxia in left upper and lower limbs that improved in a few days
-	63	THERAPEUTIC (Endoscopic Cordotomy)	Oncologic pain left arm due to breast cancer	Percutaneous endoscopic cordotomy C1-C2 with 17G needle in the right side	Viewed spinal cord, dentate ligament, spinal anterior roots.	Satisfactory control of pain

Using our proposed double-channel micro-endoscopic percutaneous cordotomy technique, we could simultaneously visualize the target point on the spinal cord and the radiofrequency (RF) probe in 91.7% of cases (Fig. **5**). In two instances, the single-channel technique was sufficient to complete the procedure. Cordotomy resulted in adequate pain control, with excellent short-term outcomes; however, pain recurrence may occur due to disease progression. Patients tolerated the procedure well, with the most common complaint being mild headaches during the immediate postoperative period. Two patients experienced significant ataxia, which ultimately resolved within a few weeks. There were no cerebrospinal fluid (CSF) leaks, permanent morbidity, or intraoperative/postoperative mortality [11, 12].

DISCUSSION

In 1931, Burman [4] pioneered myeloscopy, facilitating the direct examination of the spinal cord (SC). This innovation was subsequently complemented by Pool's delineation of intrathecal endoscopy in 1942, wherein he chronicled outcomes from an extensive series of over 400 myeloscopic interventions. Yet, the allure of myeloscopy waned, primarily attributed to morbidities linked with the introduction of a substantial bore scope into the spinal canal. Presently, endoscopic techniques have become ubiquitous for executing minimally invasive interventions within the epidural domain, including discectomies pertaining to disc herniations [5].

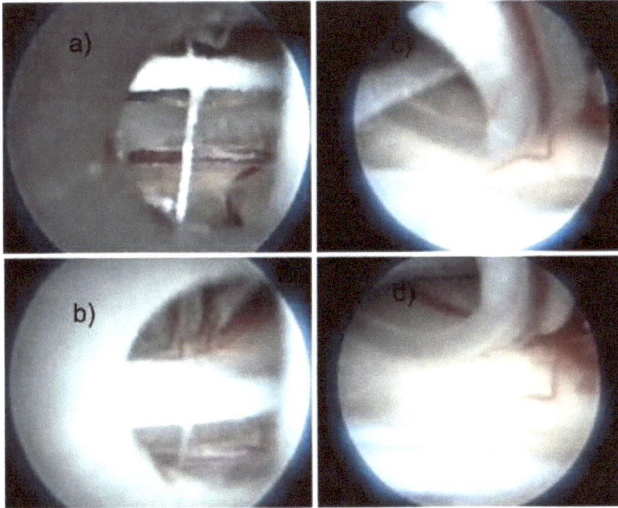

Fig. (5). *via* an endoscopic approach, a clear visualization of the intradural expanse within the spinal canal is achieved. This apparatus proffers a 70° visual field (a, b) with 40X magnification, aligned at a 0° observational angle (d,c). Endoscopic imagery, procured intraoperatively, facilitates the identification of the intradural medulla along with the rootlet origins. Subsequent to precise electrical neurostimulation confirming the implicated nerve root, radiofrequency ablation was judiciously executed.

Years later, in 1974, Olinger and Ohlhaber [6, 7] conceived a slender fiberoptic needle endoscope, narrow enough to navigate through a 17-gauge spinal needle. This apparatus was employed to visualize the craniocervical junction during medullary procedures. Notwithstanding the absence of transformative surgical breakthroughs at that time, they postulated prospective applications of such instrumentation for intraspinal operations, proffering direct inspection *via* constricted access points.

Historically, cordotomies were predominantly carried out utilizing open laminectomy at thoracic segments or, alternatively, percutaneous approaches at upper cervical strata, leveraging indirect observation grounded on fluoroscopic oleaginous contrast myelography, a technique articulated by Mullan and Rosomoff [8]. The percutaneous radiofrequency paradigm has since become the favored methodology, and has demonstrated consistent success at our own surgical establishment since the 1970s. Nonetheless, this modality necessitates an adept surgical hand capable of discerning occasionally ambiguous myelographic portrayals. Furthermore, the application of oleaginous contrast mediums poses the risk of engendering arachnoiditis and exhibits prolonged retention within the cerebrospinal milieu [9].

A more recent advance in cordotomy involves CT-based myelography guidance [10]. However, this technique presents challenges, as it requires the injection of contrast material into the spinal canal, and relies on access to a computerized tomography scanner, which is not typically available in the operating rooms of most healthcare institutions. The success and complication rates associated with cordotomy primarily hinge on the precise placement of the radiofrequency electrode, given that the lesions created through this approach are localized. Directly visualizing anatomical landmarks during the procedure enhances the surgeon's ability to identify the target site accurately, thus improving overall safety. Additionally, the new endoscopic technique offers several advantages, including shorter procedure times, reduced reliance on fluoroscopy, and eliminating contrast agents. These advancements hold promise for advancing the field of spinal interventions.

CONCLUSION

At present, intradural spinal endoscopy offers a safer approach for manipulating nervous tissue than surgical procedures. New holder devices have been developed to secure the endoscope in place, allowing the insertion of additional instruments for precise handling of neural tissue or treatment of other lesions. This advancement opens up new possibilities for minimally invasive spinal interventions, reducing the risks associated with traditional surgical approaches, and potentially improving cancer patient outcomes by reducing resistant pain.

REFERENCES

[1]   Deandrea S, Corli O, Consonni D, Villani W, Greco MT, Apolone G. Prevalence of breakthrough cancer pain: a systematic review and a pooled analysis of published literature. J Pain Symptom Manage 2014; 47(1): 57-76.
[http://dx.doi.org/10.1016/j.jpainsymman.2013.02.015] [PMID: 23796584]

[2]   Avellanal M, Diaz-Reganon G, Orts A, Gonzalez-Montero L, Riquelme I. Transforaminal Epiduroscopy in Patients with Failed Back Surgery Syndrome. Pain Physician 2019; 1(22;1): 89-95.
[http://dx.doi.org/10.36076/ppj/2019.22.89] [PMID: 30700072]

[3]   Avellanal M, Diaz-Reganon G. Interlaminar approach for epiduroscopy in patients with failed back surgery syndrome. Br J Anaesth 2008; 101(2): 244-9.
[http://dx.doi.org/10.1093/bja/aen165] [PMID: 18552347]

[4]   MS B. Myeloscopy or the direct visualization of the spinal cord and its contents. JBJS 1931; 13: 695-6.

[5]   Ruetten S, Komp M, Merk H, Godolias G. Full-endoscopic cervical posterior foraminotomy for the operation of lateral disc herniations using 5.9-mm endoscopes: a prospective, randomized, controlled study. Spine 2008; 33(9): 940-8.
[http://dx.doi.org/10.1097/BRS.0b013e31816c8b67] [PMID: 18427313]

[6]   Olinger CP, Ohlhaber RL. Eighteen-gauge needle endoscope with flexible viewing system. Surg Neurol 1975; 4(6): 537-8.
[PMID: 1188594]

[7]   Olinger CP, Ohlhaber RL. Eighteen-gauge microscopic-telescopic needle endoscope with electrode channel: potential clinical and research application. Surg Neurol 1974; 2(3): 151-60.
[PMID: 4829029]

[8]   Mullan S. Percutaneous Cordotomy. J Neurosurg 1971; 35(3): 360-6.
[http://dx.doi.org/10.3171/jns.1971.35.3.0360] [PMID: 22046654]

[9]   Hwang SW, Bhadelia RA, Wu J. Thoracic spinal iophendylate-induced arachnoiditis mimicking an intramedullary spinal cord neoplasm. J Neurosurg Spine 2008; 8(3): 292-4.
[http://dx.doi.org/10.3171/SPI/2008/8/3/292] [PMID: 18312083]

[10]   Kanpolat Y, Ugur HC, Ayten M, Elhan AH. Computed tomography-guided percutaneous cordotomy for intractable pain in malignancy. Neurosurgery 2009; 64(3) (Suppl.): ons187-93.
[PMID: 19240568]

[11]   Fonoff ET, Lopez WOC, de Oliveira YSA, Teixeira MJ. Microendoscopy-guided percutaneous cordotomy for intractable pain: case series of 24 patients. J Neurosurg 2016; 124(2): 389-96.
[http://dx.doi.org/10.3171/2014.12.JNS141616] [PMID: 26230468]

[12]   Fonoff ET, de Oliveira YSA, Lopez WOC, Alho EJL, Lara NA, Teixeira MJ. Endoscopic-guided percutaneous radiofrequency cordotomy. J Neurosurg 2010; 113(3): 524-7.
[http://dx.doi.org/10.3171/2010.4.JNS091779] [PMID: 20433282]

CHAPTER 7

Endoscopic Anatomy of the Transcallosal Hemispherotomy: A Cadaver Study With Advanced 3D Modeling

René O. Varela[1,*], Alberto Di Somma[2], Jose Pineda[3], Pedro Roldán[4], Jordi Rumià[4], Alberto G. Prats[3] and William Omar Contreras López[5]

[1] *Department of Neurosurgery, Universidad del Valle, Instituto Neurológico del Pacífico, Valle del Cauca, Colombia*

[2] *Division of Neurosurgery, Department of Neurosciences, Reproductive and Odontostomatological Sciences, Università degli Studi di Napoli Federico II, Napoles, Italy*

[3] *Laboratory of Surgical Neuroanatomy, Faculty of Medicine, Universidad de Barcelona, Barcelona, Spain*

[4] *Department of Neurosurgery, Hospital Clinic, Faculty of Medicine, Universidad de Barcelona, Barcelona, Spain*

[5] *Clínica Foscal Internacional, Autopista Floridablanca - Girón, Km 7, Floridablanca, Santander, Colombia*

Abstract: Transcallosal hemispherotomy is a surgical procedure used to treat severe epileptic seizures from a single brain hemisphere. This procedure involves the disconnection of the affected hemisphere from the rest of the brain, effectively preventing the spread of epileptic activity and reducing the frequency and severity of seizures. Endoscopic anatomy plays a crucial role in transcallosal hemispherectomy, as it allows for a minimally invasive approach. Using endoscopic techniques, surgeons can access and visualize the corpus callosum, a thick bundle of nerve fibers connecting the two cerebral hemispheres. This technique provides a clear view of the anatomical landmarks and enables precise disconnection of the affected hemisphere, while preserving critical neural structures. In this chapter, the authors review the endoscopic anatomy relevant to the transcallosal hemispherectomy identification of the corpus callosum's rostrum, genu, body, and splenium. By carefully navigating through these structures, surgeons can safely sever the connections between the affected and healthy hemispheres. This disconnection allows for better seizure control and improved quality of life for patients with severe epilepsy. The use of an endoscopic technique for transcallosal hemispherectomy may enable neurosurgeons to employ a minimally invasive approach to accomplish a precise disconnection of the affected hemisphere. It may thus form the basis for improved patient outcomes.

* Corresponding autor René O. Varela: Department of Neurosurgery, Universidad del Valle, Instituto Neurológico del Pacífico, Valle del Cauca, Colombia; E-mail: renevarelaosorio@me.com

Keywords: Anatomical landmarks, Endoscopic technique, Epileptic seizures, Transcallosal hemispherotomy.

INTRODUCTION

Hemispheric epileptic perturbations frequently culminate in calamitous seizure syndromes, predominantly manifesting in pediatric cohorts. In pediatric patients with refractory epilepsy, surgical intervention stands as a pivotal therapeutic avenue, yielding favorable results with judicious candidate selection [1 - 3]. Traditional disconnective modalities, like callosotomy, have conventionally been executed *via* expansive craniotomies utilizing microscopic guidance [4, 5]. These operative techniques, however, can engender complications; including augmented hemodynamic perturbations, intensified postsurgical discomfort, and concomitant protraction of hospitalization durations [6 - 8]. The refinement of microsurgical techniques [1, 4, 5] and improvements in instrumentation, imaging, robotics [9], and surgical image guidance systems [4, 10] facilitated the use of more minimally invasive approaches and surgical techniques in neurosurgery [11, 12]. These endoscopic techniques are gaining popularity as their application in functional neurosurgery has demonstrated that the endoscope can be used as a valuable tool to perform disconnective procedures in a minimally invasive fashion [11, 13]. While the surgical steps and clinical outcomes are similar to those used in microsurgical techniques, fewer complications have been noted [14, 15]. In this chapter, the authors undertake a detailed description of the intracerebral architecture, as approached through an endoscopic transcallosal conduit. To this end, they conducted a cadaveric examination of the pertinent surgical topography, providing a methodical exposition of the endoscopic transcallosal hemispherotomy procedure. Additionally, the authors present a 3D modeling analysis of the surgical anatomy to help the prospective endoscopic neurosurgeon better understand the complex anatomy of the endoscopic transcallosal hemispherotomy.

Historical Perspectives

In 1928, Dandy pioneered the anatomical hemispherectomy for addressing hemispheric epilepsy, specifically targeting infiltrating gliomas in the non-dominant hemisphere [16]. This groundbreaking surgical intervention entailed a comprehensive excision of a cerebral hemisphere inclusive of the basal ganglia, in conjunction with the severance of both the anterior and middle cerebral arteries post-bifurcation. The resultant surgical tableau revealed the corpus callosum, falx cerebri, tentorium, and the olfactory and optic nerves at the cranial base. A subsequent iteration by Gardner [17] retained the basal ganglia, cleaving the anterior and middle cerebral arteries subsequent to the genesis of the deep perforators. This adaptation heralded enhanced postoperative motor prognoses concurrent with successful seizure management. McKenzie, in 1938, employed this procedure in a Canadian context for epilepsy treatment, specifically targeting infantile hemiplegia cases [18]. The adoption of the procedure continued to grow post-1950, epitomized by Krynauw's documentation of 12 pediatric epilepsy cases with concomitant behavioral alterations, which post-surgery exhibited promising seizure resolutions [19]. By 1952, Penfield and Rasmussen had implemented this methodology at the Montreal Neurological Institute [17, 20, 21].

While the anatomical hemispherectomy garnered widespread endorsement, it was not devoid of complications, notably including hydrocephalus [22, 23] and superficial cerebral hemosiderosis. Notwithstanding these challenges, the technique delivered impressive seizure cessation rates ranging between 43% and 90% [24]. Evolution in surgical practices led to the conceptualization of functional hemispherectomy and, subsequently, hemispherotomy; a paradigm initially posited by Olivier Delalande, which later bifurcated into two surgical trajectories: the vertical and peri-insular approaches championed by Delalande and Villemure, respectively [2, 3, 7, 23]. Both Delalande [25] and Villemure [23] proffered hemispherotomies necessitating expansive craniotomies compared to Schramm's approach, which emphasized a diminutive cortical excision, opting instead to functionally segregate the epileptic cortex from subcortical entities [26, 27]. This revised strategy yielded exemplary results, with 75%-90% of patients attaining a seizure-free state, as well as reduced morbidity rates [21]. Subsequent scholarly assessments focused on the merits of Schramm's technique, highlighting the limited craniotomy requisites, minimal cerebral parenchyma resection, diminished postoperative hydrocephalus risk, and lesser transfusion necessities [28]. Still, the perpetual pursuit for refined, patient-centric, minimally invasive modalities with concomitant reductions in blood loss and complications catalyzed the authors' elucidation of the endoscopic hemispherotomy technique, an exemplar of which is elaborated below.

Pre-dissection Planning and Quantitative Protocol

First, the authors set up the dissection limits of our functional disconnection. To this end, critical intracranial landmarks were selected, and the following were taken into account:

1. Genu of the corpus callosum, in its most anterior extreme,
2. Tentorium (tentorial apex),
3. Atrium of the lateral ventricle, in the glomus of the Choroid plexus,
4. Temporal ventricle horn

Based upon the above anatomic references, we categorized the hemispherical disconnection into five main steps:

1. Corpus callosotomy,
2. Anterior frontal-basal disconnection,
3. Posterior disconnection,
4. Lateral disconnection,
5. Hippocampal disconnection

The following relevant anatomic measurements were drawn from the pre-surgical MRI scans:

1. Distance between anterior and posterior edges of the craniotomy,
2. Distance between lateral and medial edges of the craniotomy,
3. Distance between the coronal suture and the anterior commissure,
4. Distance between the coronal suture and the corpus callosum, using a line between the coronal suture and the anterior commissure as a reference,
5. Distance between the anterior edge of the craniotomy and the Genu,
6. Distance between the posterior edge of the craniotomy and the Splenium,
7. Distance between the Genu (the most anterior part of the corpus callosum) and the Splenium (the most posterior part of the corpus callosum),
8. Distance between the coronal suture and temporal horn,
9. Distance between the temporal horn and middle cerebral artery bifurcation
10. The angle between the anterior edge of the craniotomy and the most anterior part of the Genu,
11. The angle between the posterior edge of the craniotomy and the most posterior part of the Splenium,
12. The angle between the lateral edge of the craniotomy at the level of the coronal suture and temporal horn

Measurement of each disconnection was also performed (the callosotomy and the anterior, lateral, posterior, and hippocampal disconnections) as follows:

1. Callosotomy: the distance between the Genu (the most anterior part of the corpus callosum) and the Splenium (the most posterior part of the corpus callosum),
2. Anterior disconnection: the distance between a point on the gyrus rectus (at the anterior skull base, level of the most anterior part of the Genu on the midline) and the middle cerebral artery bifurcation,
3. Lateral disconnection: the distance between a point in the Atrium (glomus) and another at the frontal horn,

4. Posterior disconnection: the distance between a point located at the most posterior and inferior part of the Splenium and another point located on the fornix at the level of the thalamus' Pulvinar,

5. Hippocampal disconnection: the distance between a point located on the posterior hippocampus (at the level of the intermolecular line) and another point located on the most medial part of the temporal horn (bordering the superior and lateral surface of the hippocampus).

The descriptive and regression statistical analyses were carried out using STATA 14. Several variables were analyzed, including the mean of the distances between anatomical structures and the disconnection lengths. Linear regression was performed between corpus callosum disconnection and the Genu – Splenium distance.

Anatomic Dissections and 3D Modeling

Anatomical explorations and dissections were performed at the Laboratory of Surgical Neuroanatomy (LSNA) within the Human Anatomy and Embryology Unit at the University of Barcelona, Spain. Six cadaveric heads, translating to 12 hemispheres, were employed in this research, each with a red latex-infused arterial system. The University of Barcelona's Institutional Review Board approved this scholarly endeavor. Advanced multi-slice helical CT imaging (Siemens SOMATOM Sensation 64, Malvern, PA) was carried out, employing 0.6 mm axial spiral sections and a 0° gantry angle, both pre- and post-dissection. Complementarily, 3T MRIs were conducted to corroborate accurate disconnections, following an analogous dissection protocol. Fusion techniques juxtaposing pre- and post-disconnection MRI facilitated a key quantitative assessment. Critical markers, congruent with both CT and MRI, were permanently engrafted into the specimens' cranial structures, bolstering co-registration with the neuronavigation apparatus (Medtronic®, Louisville, KY, USA). Imaging repositories were seamlessly transitioned to the navigation-centric laboratory workstation, wherein point registration protocols stipulated a permissible deviation margin of 2 mm.

For the disconnective technique, a specialized rigid endoscope, characterized by its 4 mm diameter, 18 cm length, and dual-lens (0-degree and 30-degree) capabilities was employed (Karl *et al.*). This endoscopic conduit was interfaced with a luminous 300 W Xenon source (Karl Storz) *via* an optical fiber tether and terminated in an HD visualization node (Endovision®; Karl Storz). Preliminary microsurgical delineations, indicating the procedural trajectory, benefitted from magnification gradients spanning 3x to 40x (OPMI; Zeiss *et al.*). The procedure entailed the cadaveric specimen being positioned in a modulated supine orientation, marginally flexed to approximately 15°. Subsequent to a strategically contoured horseshoe epidermal incision, informed by the juxtaposition of coronal and sagittal sutures, a 3 x 1.5 cm craniotomy was performed under the guidance of the neuronavigation platform. Distinctive frontal and parietal parasagittal perforations were formed through meticulous high-velocity drilling, adhering to specific locational coordinates. The subsequent dural aperture and medial retraction were followed by the endoscope's introduction, mirroring the surgical tenets set forth by Chandra *et al.* in their endoscopy-assisted interhemispheric transcallosal hemispherotomy [14]. Five procedural segments encapsulated the hemispherotomy, each meticulously rendered *via* dedicated three-dimensional simulations to maximize comprehension. This immersive 3D topography, sculpted utilizing Amira 3D for Life Sciences (ThermoFisher® *et al.*, Oregon, USA), integrated precisely segmented bony constituents and clearly demarcated surgical purview territories, facilitated by the advanced analytical capabilities of the Amira workstation.

Endoscopic Transcallosal Hemispherotomy

Craniotomy and Durotomy

In this meticulous dissection, the authors executed an endoscopic hemispherotomy on all the cadaveric specimens, leveraging a minimalistic craniotomy approach, while carefully averting damage to the proximate vascular architecture of each cerebral hemisphere. Upon dural incision, a profusion of arachnoid adhesions, ensconced between the hemisphere's medial facet and the falx, were cautiously severed. The Callosomarginal artery, intricately linked with the cingulate sulcus, was the first structure unveiled, often emanating from the pericallosal artery in tandem with the pericallosal cistern. Both pericallosal conduits were carefully preserved and laterally redirected towards the midline, culminating in the revelation of the corpus callosum. The endoscope was precisely navigated into the interstice demarcated by the falx and the cerebral matter (Refer to Fig. **1**).

Callosotomy

After obtaining optimal visualization of the corpus callosum, dissection is pursued anteriorly along its vertical plane until the genu becomes discernible. For clear visualization of the splenium and tentorium, respectively, the optimal angulations are 50.2° proximal to the anterior boundary of the craniotomy and 60.4° relative to its posterior boundary. The endoscope is subsequently navigated toward the anterior segment of the corpus callosum, meticulously parsing numerous arachnoid membranes and demarcating the arterial ensemble comprised of the anterior cerebral artery, gyrus cingulum, and the peri-callosal mustache adjoined beneath. Precise identification and cautious dissection of the gyrus cingulum are paramount to avoid any inadvertent damage. The pericallosal arteries are strategically displaced laterally adjacent to the midline, providing unobstructed exposure of the corpus callosum (Fig. **2**). Upon fully exposing the corpus callosum, extending from the genu to the splenium, callosotomy is executed marginally lateral to the midline on the congruent side of disconnection. Initially, the anterior segment is cleaved, facilitating entry into the ventricular system. Subsequently, landmarks such as the foramen of Monro and the choroid plexus are identified. The caudate nucleus' head, positioned superiorly and laterally on the frontal horn's lateral wall, is then discerned (Fig. **2**).

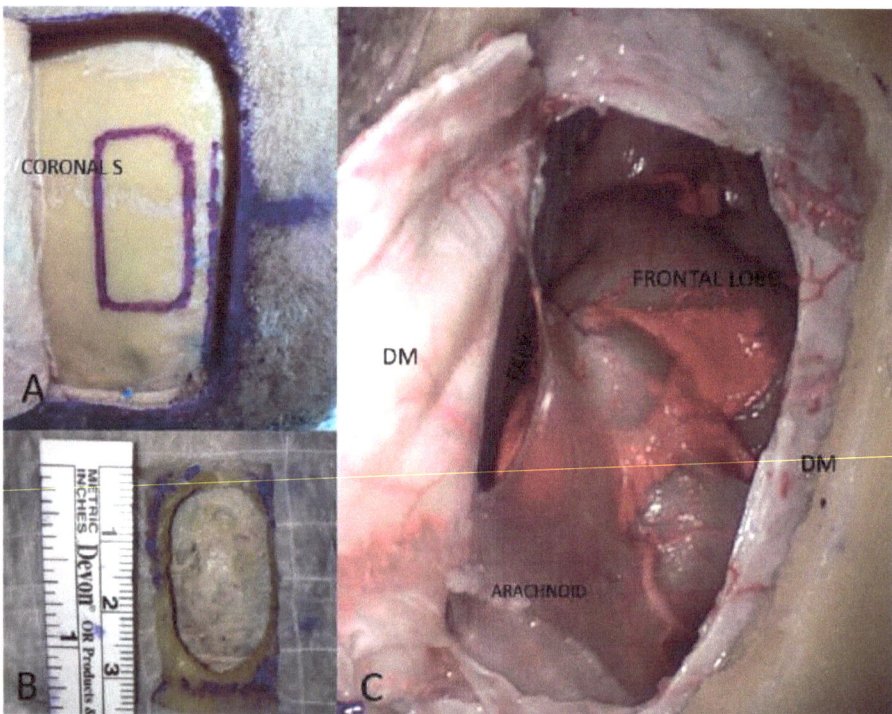

Fig. (1). A) Craniotomy Dimensions: A precise 3 x 1.5 cm craniotomy was executed. **B)** Anatomical Landmarks for Craniotomy: Positioned 1 cm anteriorly and 2 cm posteriorly relative to the coronal suture, and only 0.5 cm laterally from the central axis. **C)** Dural Incision and Endoscopic Insertion: The dura mater was incised in a C-configured manner, subsequently reflected towards the medial aspect. The endoscope was introduced into the space delineated by the falx and cerebral tissue. Abbreviations: CORONAL S = Coronal Suture; DM = Dura Mater.

The systematic procedure for endoscopic callosotomy is delineated as follows: Initially, the pericallosal arteries are shifted laterally adjacent to the midline, accompanied by gentle cerebral retraction. Callosotomy commences at the anterior tertile, progressing towards the genu. The frontal horn comes into view, with the caudate nucleus' head identified laterally. Pursuing the curvature of the anterior cerebral artery, the callosotomy reaches the genu, ensuring its comprehensive disconnection up to the subcallosal gyrus. The dissection continues posteriorly, culminating at the divided splenium. Upon cleavage of the splenium, entry into the lateral ventricle's atrium is achieved, marking the completion of the corpus callosotomy.

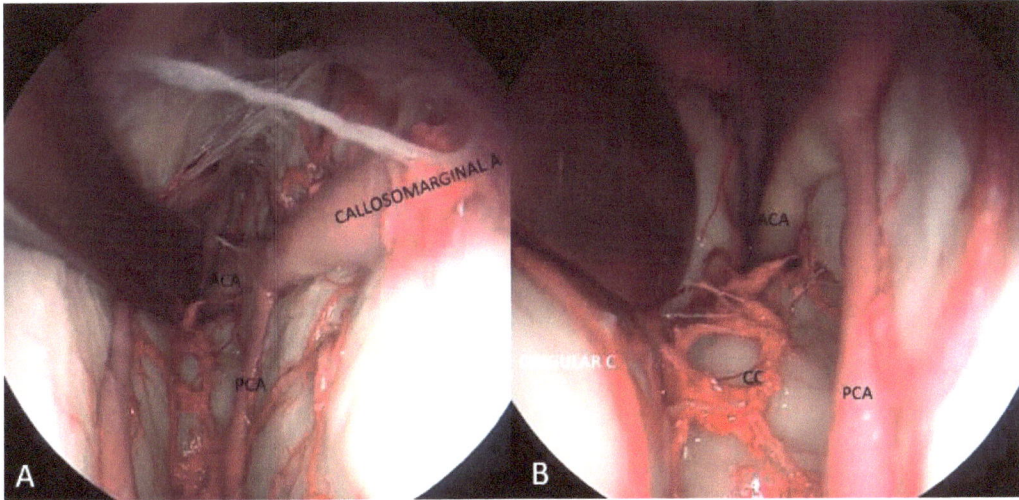

Fig. (2). Endoscopic Visualization Along the Parasagittal Plane of the Corpus Callosum. (**A**) With the endoscope strategically positioned toward the anterior segment of the corpus callosum, intricate dissections of the principal arachnoid membranes are conducted, elucidating the arterial architecture of the A.C.A., the intricacies of the gyrus cingulum, and the details of the pericallosal mustache nestled below. (**B**) Precision in identifying and meticulous dissection of the gyrus cingulum is imperative to mitigate potential damage. The pericallosal arteries are repositioned laterally, adjacent to the midline, rendering an unobstructed view of the corpus callosum. Abbreviations: A.C.A. = Anterior Cerebral Artery; CALLOSOMARGINAL A = Callosomarginal Artery; CC = Corpus Callosum; CINGULAR G = Cingular Gyrus; P.C.A. = Pericallosal Artery.

In this phase, anatomical verification was ascertained by tracing the inferior margin of the falx cerebri. This meanders inferiorly posterior to the splenium, facilitating the identification of the tentorial apex, and subsequently revealing the Galen vein and the internal cerebral veins beneath the arachnoid membrane. Progression in the disconnection of the genu persisted until the subcallosal gyrus came into view. The subsequent callosotomy advanced in the direction of the splenium, bifurcating it and further delineating the tentorial apex. Upon the culmination of the splenial division, both the atrium and glomus were discernible (Fig. **3**). These procedural nuances are depicted on representative axial T2-weighted MRI scans of a specimen from the authors' research (Fig. **4**). The quantitative evaluation indicated an average corpus callosotomy extent of 90.8 mm ± 2.7 mm.

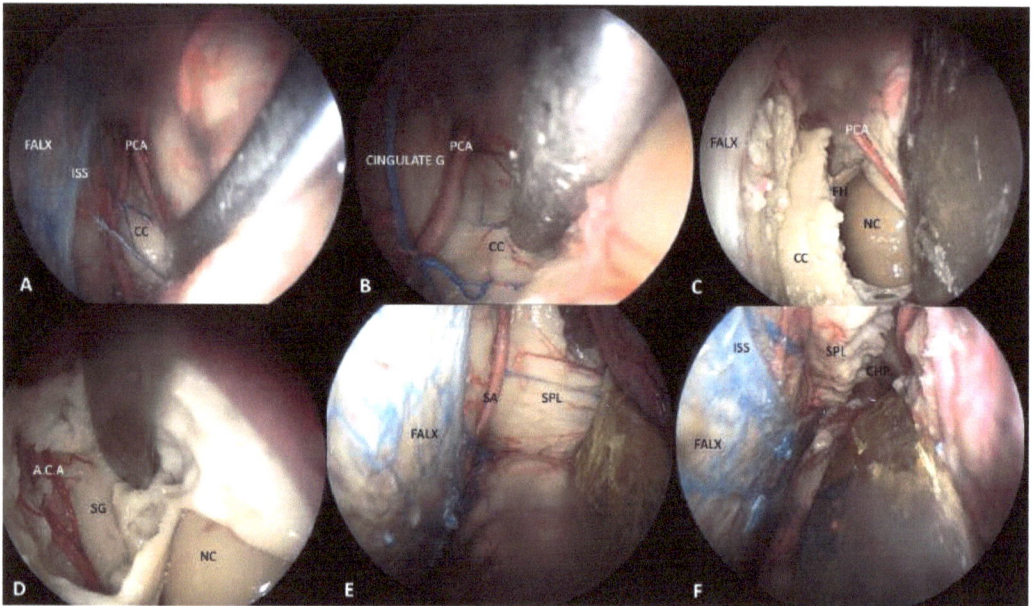

Fig. (3). Endoscopic Callosotomy Procedure: (**A**) Initiate by laterally diverting the pericallosal arteries from the midline, followed by a delicate cerebral retraction. (**B**) Callosotomy is initiated anteriorly, progressing directly towards the genu. (**C**) The frontal horn is brought into the visual field, revealing the lateral position of the nucleus caudate's head. (**D**) Continue the disconnection until the subcallosal gyrus emerges into view. (**E**) Progressing the callosotomy towards the splenium facilitates the revelation of the tentorial apex. (**F**) Upon complete splenial division, both the atrium and glomus become discernible. Abbreviations: CHP = Choroidal Plexus; FH = Frontal Horn; ISS = Inferior Sagittal Sinus; NC = Nucleus Caudate's Head; SA = Splenial Artery; SG = Subcallosal Gyrus.

Anterior Disconnection

Sequential Anterior Disconnection Process: Upon completion of the corpus callosotomy, the anterior disconnection was initiated commencing at the subcallosal gyrus echelon. A precise corticectomy within the subcallosal cortex was executed, progressing towards the anterior cranial fossa floor until convergence with the gyrus rectus. Subsequently, the corticectomy trajectory shifted laterally, navigating anterior to the caudate nucleus's head, consistent with the lesser wing of the sphenoid, or more precisely, the Sylvian fissure's nascent section. This phase permitted visualization of structures encompassing the olfactory tract, the inaugural segment of the anterior cerebral arteries, the internal carotid bifurcation, and the optic nerve's terminal segment; all delineated through the arachnoid. Additionally, the middle cerebral artery's course could be discerned from its proximal to distal extents. This anterior disconnection abrogates connective pathways originating from the anterior temporal lobe, amygdala, and frontal lobe (Fig. **5**). The quantitative assessment indicated the mean span of this disconnection to be approximately 43.3 mm ± 3.5 mm.

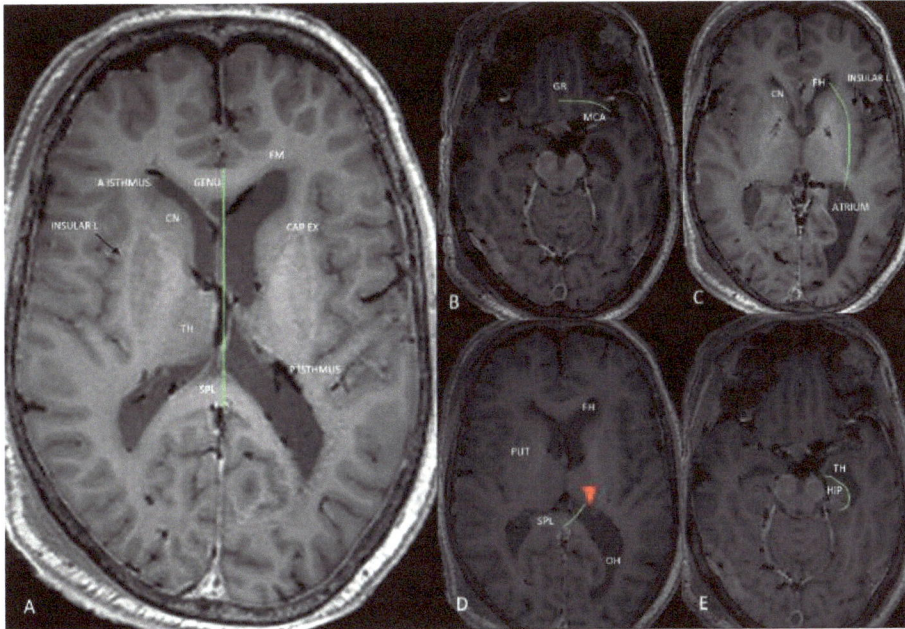

Fig. (4). Illustration of the Sequential Disconnection Procedure: (**A**) The callosotomy was initiated at the anterior segment of the corpus callosum, advancing through the genu and culminating posteriorly at the splenium. (**B**) Anterior dissection commenced post-genu partitioning, extending towards the anterior cranial fossa floor, ultimately targeting the gyrus rectus inferiorly, with an aim to localize the MCA. (**C**) The lateral disconnection bridges the anterior and posterior isthmus, encompassing the external capsule, claustrum, and extrema complex. (**D**) Posterior disconnection seeks to access the choroidal fissure, consequently disrupting the fornix continuity. (**E**) Disconnection of the hippocampus was meticulously executed, encompassing its lateral contour. *Abbreviations*: A ISTHMUS = Anterior Isthmus; CAP EXT = Capsule externe; CN = Caudate nucleus; FM = Forceps major; FH = Frontal horn; GR = Gyrus rectus; HIP = Hippocampus; INSULAR L = Insular lobe; MCA = Middle cerebral artery; OH = Occipital horn; PUT = Putamen; SPL = Splenium; TH = Thalamus.

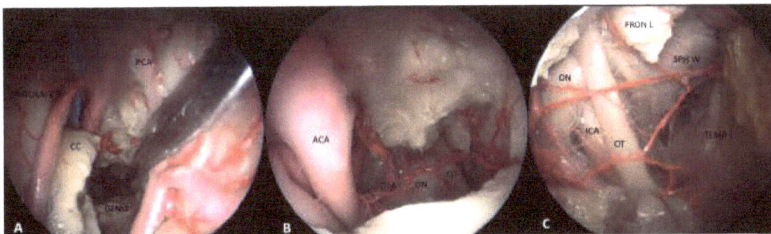

Fig. (5). Anterior Disconnection: (**A**) The anterior disconnection is carried out after the complete callosotomy until it reaches the floor of the anterior skull base. (**B**) The disconnection is directed laterally to the lesser sphenoid wing passing anteriorly to the head of the caudate nucleus. (**C**) The anterior cerebral arteries (ACA), the olfactory tract, the carotid, internal bifurcation, and the distal part of the optic nerve can be visualized through the arachnoid. *Abbreviations:* FRON L = Frontal lobe; ICA = Internal carotid artery; OFA = Orbitofrontal artery; ON = Optic nerve; OT = Olfactory tract; SPH W = Lesser sphenoid wing; TEMP L = Temporal lobe.

Posterior Disconnection

Upon finalizing the anterior disengagement, the posterior detachment was conducted, involving the severance of the fornix's posterior column within the collateral trigone. Every crus of the fornix emerges as an extension from the fimbria, navigating between the choroidal fissure and the pulvinar's posterior facet of the thalamus, subsequently integrating into the splenium's inferior and posterior regions (Fig. **6**). This succinct disconnection spanned an approximate length of 15.7 mm ± 2.2 mm.

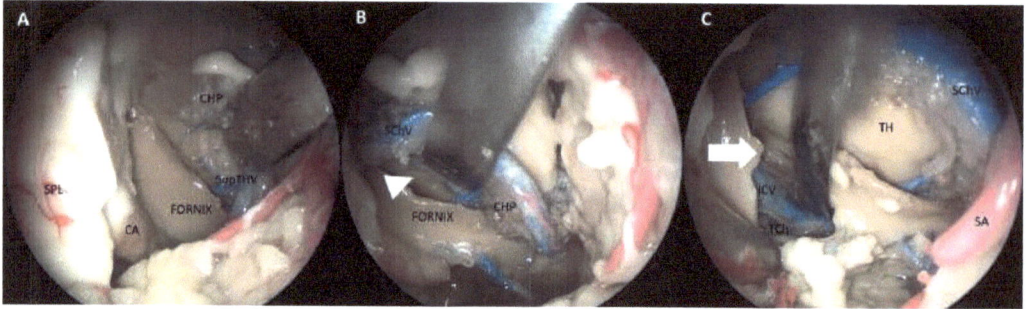

Fig. (6). Posterior Disconnection Process: (**A**) Upon detaching the splenium, (**B**) notable structures such as the atrium of the lateral ventricle, fornix, choroid plexus, and choroidal fissure become evident. A slender interstice situated between the fornix and the thalamus, spanning the medial section of the body, atrium, and temporal horn, is revealed (denoted by arrowhead in B). (**C**) The core of the posterior disconnection lies in severing the posterior column of the fornix at the collateral trigone, aiming for congruence. The splenium's separation is demarcated by the white arrow. Originating anterior to the velum interpositum, the internal cerebral veins lie just posterior to the foramen of Monro. Abbreviations: CA = Calcar Avis; CHP = Choroidal plexus; ICV = Internal cerebral vein; SA = Splenial artery; SChV = Superior Choroidal Vein; SPL = Splenium; SupTHV = Superior Thalamic vein; TCh = Tela Choroidea (upper wall); TH = Thalamus.

Lateral Disconnection

Initiating anteriorly, the lateral disengagement progressed by segmenting the thalamus as the choroidal plexus transitioned from the foramen of Monro towards the temporal horn, proceeding laterally to the lenticular nucleus. This path was delineated between the basal ganglia and insula until it converged with the anterior isthmus. Subsequently, the temporal horn's linkage to the lateral ventricle's body *via* the spinothalamic sulcus could be severed by amalgamating the lateral and anterior disjunctions. During this phase, the middle cerebral artery emerges in the anterior-inferior facet of the disconnection. Surgically, this segment severs connections encompassing the amygdala, hippocampus, fibers emanating from the occipito-parietal region, insular cortex, the bulk of the projection fibers stemming from the frontotemporal lobe, and anterior temporal junctions. The average span of this lateral detachment was noted to be 73.5 mm ± 1.26 mm (Fig. **7**).

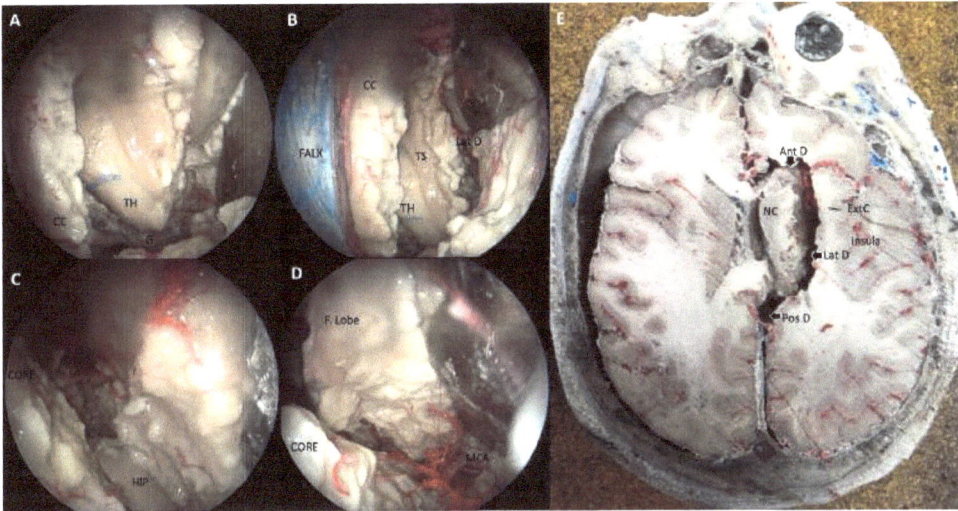

Fig. (7). Lateral Disengagement: (**A**) Initiated lateral to the glomus, and advancing anteriorly to segregate the thalamus and basal ganglia from the insular cortex, culminating at the anterior isthmus. (**B**) The strategy involves meticulous dissection between the central structure and the insular cortex, with a focus on cleaving through the white matter tracts. (**C**) Within this lateral disengagement trajectory, the ceiling of the temporal horn is discernible, with the hippocampus situated inferiorly. (**D**) At the confluence of the lateral and anterior disengagements, the middle cerebral artery becomes evident at the nadir of the separation. This juncture signifies the transition from the basal facet of the frontal lobe to the apex of the temporal lobe, located slightly posterior to the sphenoid ridge. (**E**) An axial section of the cranium illustrates the anterior, posterior, and lateral disengagements. Abbreviations: Ant D = Anterior Disengagement; CC = Corpus Callosum; Ext C = External Capsule; F. Lobe = Frontal Lobe; G = Glomus; HIP = Hippocampus; Lat D = Lateral Disengagement; MCA = Middle Cerebral Artery; NC = Caudate Nucleus Head; Pos D = Posterior Disengagement; TH = Thalamus; TS = Terminal Stria.

Hippocampal Disconnection

Upon incising the temporal apex, visual access to the hippocampus, the anterior protuberance of the amygdala, and the fimbria is attained. The disengagement was methodically executed along the hippocampus's lateral aspect *via* the collateral sulcus, encompassing both the hippocampal head and its posterior region near the lateral mesencephalic notch. Seizure-propagating longitudinal fibers were also incised. The average extent of this hippocampal disengagement was measured to be 39.1 mm ± 3.4 mm (Fig. **8**).

The Endoscopic Innovation

Within academic circles, there exist very few articles addressing endoscopic hemispherectomy in cadaveric specimens. Bahuleyan *et al.* [11] described an endoscopic trans-ventricular hemispherotomy technique. This approach, however, entailed employing both anterior and posterior burr holes, devoid of a neuronavigation system and was executed *via* dual routes. Such a modality might pose challenges in instances of small ventricles. Consequently, the present study's authors were motivated to devise a streamlined, minimally invasive singular-access corridor, leveraging cutting-edge endoscopic innovations. In 2015, Chandra *et al.* [14] published a seminal work detailing endoscopy-assisted interhemispheric transcallosal hemispherotomy performed on 11 primarily pediatric patients, boasting well-defined criteria: a remarkable 81.1% exhibited Engel's Class I outcomes. Sood *et al.* [15] carried out a posterior interhemispheric strategy, augmenting it with an endoscope fitted with suction, and employing a bimanual technique. Two pediatric subjects treated this way demonstrated seizure cessation and MRI evidence of total disconnection.

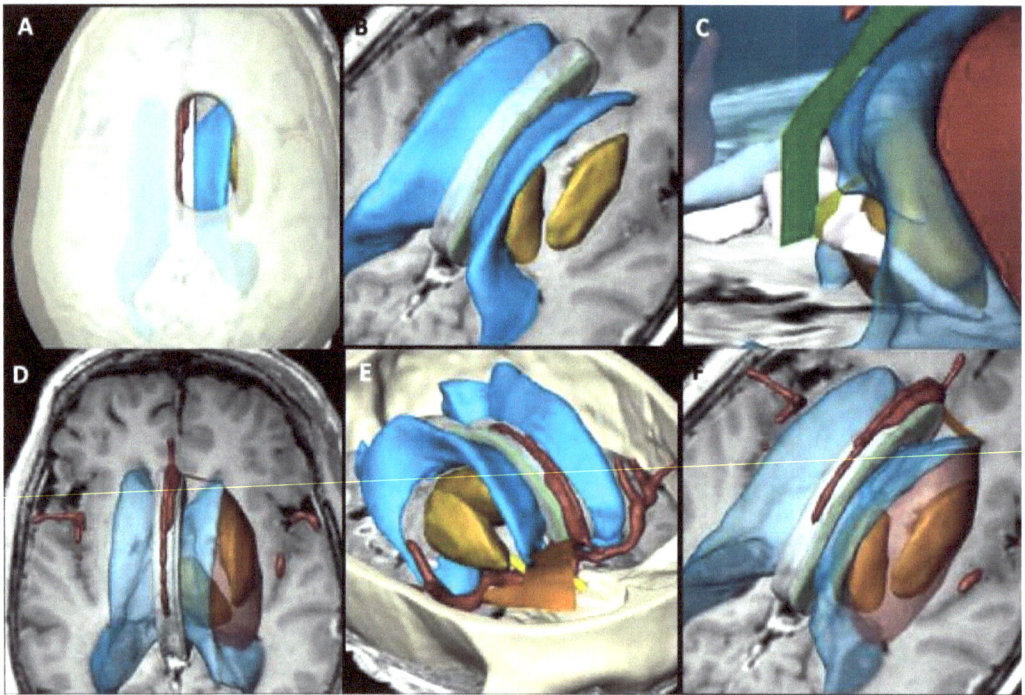

Fig. (8). 3D Anatomical Visualization of Endoscopic Transcallosal Hemispherotomy: A virtual three-dimensional representation was crafted utilizing the Amira 3D software tailored for life sciences (ThermoFisher®, Oregon, USA). Osteological structures underwent segmentation, while the extents of surgical freedom were delineated using the advanced measurement and quantification tools of the Amira workstation. Presented illustrations include (**A**) Craniotomy procedure, (**B**) Endoscopic callosotomy approach, (**C**) Posterior anatomical disconnection, (**D**) Lateral anatomical separation, (**E**) Anterior anatomical disengagement, and (**F**) Amira-based reconstruction of the disconnections.

Our endoscopic methodology takes its foundation from the vertical hemispherectomy as postulated by Delalande. This approach has garnered considerable endorsement, even for patients without cerebral atrophy, such as those with hemimegalencephaly, as evidenced by a patient series demonstrating favorable seizure results. A few scholars advocate for the excision of a segment of the superior frontal gyrus. It is imperative to acknowledge that, especially in cases such as hemimegalencephaly and hemispheric dysplasia, that cerebral midlines may not coincide with cranial midlines. Consequently, Delalande *et al.* [27] identified several reliable anatomical landmarks, including the falx cerebri positioned posteriorly, the temporal horn's rooftop laterally, and the pericallosal arteries anteriorly; especially in scenarios presenting pronounced anatomical aberrations. While dissecting the interhemispheric fissure in atrophied brains proves straightforward, the technique can be labor-intensive.

DISCUSSION

The brain's commissural structures facilitate functional integration between hemispheres. The intention behind hemispherectomy is to sever the commissural and projection bundles, intercepting epileptic activity propagation to the contralateral hemisphere and the central core *via* these conduits and the limbic pathway. Notable commissural fibers include the corpus callosum and anterior commissure, while projection fibers encompass the fornix, optic and auditory radiations, and the internal capsule (Cortico-spinal tract).

For our methodology, we utilized a horseshoe-shaped incision, addressing the inherent thickness of cadaveric skin. However, the skin pliability of a living patient, particularly in the younger demographic, might make a parasagittal linear cut followed by a 3 x 1.5 cm craniotomy more appropriate. We eschewed cortical resection of the superior frontal gyrus, accessing the ventricular corpus *via* the interhemispheric corpus callosotomy. Given the commonality of structural cerebral aberrations and resultant atrophy in hemispherotomy candidates, ventriculomegaly often emerges, aiding in ventricular navigation and endoscopic instrument manipulation.

The tissue disconnection plane lies between the external capsule (Lenticulostriate Artery-fed) and the insular arteries-supplied regions, devoid of any anastomosis [29], ensuring minimal vascularization and consequently, reduced hemorrhagic risk. At the insula level, the uncinate fasciculus intersects the anterior-inferior part of the external capsule and claustrum, bridging the temporal and frontal lobes. Efficient insular cortex disconnection can be achieved by severing the insula-opercular fibers found in the extreme capsule outer layer along with the temporal stem, linking the anterior short gyrus and the insular pole to the inferior frontal and lateral orbital gyri [30].

The amygdala complex primarily receives afferents from the stria terminalis (along the caudate's tail) and the diagonal band of Broca. To effectively disrupt this fibrous system, the temporal horn roof adjacent to the choroid fissure, housing both the stria terminalis and anterior commissure, must be removed. The diagonal band of Broca extends over the middle cerebral artery, preceding the optic tracts; and upon anterior perforated substance corpectomy, both the anterior cerebral artery and MCA sections are exposed, distinctly revealing the amygdala. By continuing the anterior disconnection laterally to medially—from the orbital gyrus, through the olfactory tracts to the gyrus rectus—the anterior commissure becomes intrinsically severed. Despite the rigorous process, the risk of incomplete disconnection remains, which may perpetuate postoperative seizures. Our recommended hippocampal disconnection post temporal horn roof excision ensures thorough limbic system disconnection, especially vital for patients with concomitant hippocampal lesions [31].

Endoscopic transcallosal hemispherectomy offers various merits: minimized complications, swift and straightforward craniectomy, and a direct visual field. However, challenges arise from altered anatomical perspectives, deeper workspaces, and potentially circumscribed surgical agility—suggesting selectivity in patient candidacy. Addressing vascular hemorrhages amidst critical vascular structures remains paramount, possibly contingent on the space afforded by the atrophied hemisphere. Nevertheless, any discourse on the technique's pros and cons warrants extensive experiential investigation.

Cook *et al.* [32] pitted three hemispheric epilepsy management techniques against each other in 115 patients. Their findings demonstrated perioperative blood loss discrepancies: functional hemispherectomy averaged 288 ± 32 ml, while anatomical variants recorded 688 ± 90 ml losses. Additionally, the latter also necessitated prolonged hospitalizations and external ventriculostomy durations. Notably, 15-30% of peri insular hemispherectomy patients experienced recurrent seizures, challenging seizure management through augmented anticonvulsant regimes, Vagus nerve stimulation, or transitioning to anatomical hemispherectomy [33]. Kiehna *et al.* [34] determined a 9.1% recurrence rate in their hemispherectomy cohort, attributing it to incompletely severed tracts, discernible *via* MRI and DTI sequences. However, juxtaposing these modalities is beyond our study's purview, which seeks to elucidate the intricate surgical anatomy underpinning the pioneering endoscopic transcallosal hemispherectomy approach.

Our cadaveric study details the anatomical specifics of this hemispherectomy technique. Constraints stem from utilizing specimens with standard ventricular dimensions—a critical determinant for this surgical method. Furthermore, silicone-infused brain samples do not replicate the dynamic behavior of live tissues, posing inherent limitations.

With an intimate understanding of cerebral anatomy, the endoscopic approach could potentially rival microsurgical counterparts in safety and efficacy, especially for hemispheric epilepsy syndromes [7, 23]. Rigorous cadaveric practice is indispensable for mastering the surgical anatomy and the multifaceted protocol we propose. We hope to authenticate pertinent anatomic metrics from preoperative MRI scans, aiming to refine the endoscopic steps articulated in this discourse through more in-depth measures in afflicted patients.

CONCLUSION

This research underscores the imperative of judiciously advancing minimally invasive modalities for the surgical intervention of epilepsy. Its purview encompasses the treatment of hemispheric epileptic syndromes and the targeted disconnection of discrete cerebral lesions. Our cadaveric analysis posits that the endoscopic transcallosal hemispherotomy technique provides optimal visualization, and might achieve analogous disconnection outcomes to conventional strategies. This anatomical study delineates neurovascular constructs pertinent to the neurosurgical trajectory. Subsequent clinical investigations are essential to discern whether the indications for this endoscopic technique are confined to specific surgical challenges or pathologies. Minimally invasive endoscopic methodologies hold the potential to address certain limitations inherent in traditional procedures. The prime objective of this research, which drove us to intricately study the relevant surgical anatomy, is to mitigate morbidity and mortality *via* an advanced endoscopic disconnection method. Prospective advances suggest that endoscopic transcallosal hemispherotomy could be an invaluable augmentation to the repertoire of surgical interventions for epilepsy, benefiting patients grappling with intractable seizures.

REFERENCES

[1]   Daniel RT, Meagher-Villemure K, Farmer JP, Andermann F, Villemure JG. Posterior quadrantic epilepsy surgery: technical variants, surgical anatomy, and case series. Epilepsia 2007; 48(8): 1429-37.
[http://dx.doi.org/10.1111/j.1528-1167.2007.01095.x] [PMID: 17441997]

[2]   Daniel RT, Villemure JG. Hemispherotomy techniques. J Neurosurg 2003; 98(2): 438-9.
[PMID: 12593638]

[3]   Daniel RT, Villemure JG. Peri-insular hemispherotomy: potential pitfalls and avoidance of complications. Stereotact Funct Neurosurg 2003; 80(1-4): 22-7.
[http://dx.doi.org/10.1159/000075155] [PMID: 14745204]

[4]   Barrit S, Park EH, El Hadwe S, Madsen JR. Complete Corpus Callosotomy for Refractory Epilepsy in Children. World Neurosurg 2022; 164: 69.
[http://dx.doi.org/10.1016/j.wneu.2022.04.099] [PMID: 35500873]

[5]   Vaddiparti A, Huang R, Blihar D, *et al.* The Evolution of Corpus Callosotomy for Epilepsy Management. World Neurosurg 2021; 145: 455-61.
[http://dx.doi.org/10.1016/j.wneu.2020.08.178] [PMID: 32889189]

[6] Althausen A, Gleissner U, Hoppe C, *et al.* Long-term outcome of hemispheric surgery at different ages in 61 epilepsy patients. J Neurol Neurosurg Psychiatry 2013; 84(5): 529-36.
[http://dx.doi.org/10.1136/jnnp-2012-303811] [PMID: 23268362]

[7] Villemure JG, Mascott CR. Peri-insular Hemispherotomy. Neurosurgery 1995; 37(5): 975-80.
[http://dx.doi.org/10.1227/00006123-199511000-00018] [PMID: 8559348]

[8] Wessinger CM, Fendrich R, Ptito A, Villemure JG, Gazzaniga MS. Residual vision with awareness in the field contralateral to a partial or complete functional hemispherectomy. Neuropsychologia 1996; 34(11): 1129-37.
[http://dx.doi.org/10.1016/0028-3932(96)00023-1] [PMID: 8904751]

[9] Chandra PS, Doddamani R, Girishan S, *et al.* Robotic thermocoagulative hemispherotomy: concept, feasibility, outcomes, and safety of a new "bloodless" technique. J Neurosurg Pediatr 2021; 27(6): 688-99.
[http://dx.doi.org/10.3171/2020.10.PEDS20673] [PMID: 33799306]

[10] Ravindra VM, Ruggieri L, Gadgil N, *et al.* An Initial Experience of Completion Hemispherotomy *via* Magnetic Resonance-Guided Laser Interstitial Therapy. Stereotact Funct Neurosurg 2023; 101(3): 179-87.
[http://dx.doi.org/10.1159/000528452] [PMID: 37062282]

[11] Bahuleyan B, Manjila S, Robinson S, Cohen AR. Minimally invasive endoscopic transventricular hemispherotomy for medically intractable epilepsy: a new approach and cadaveric demonstration. J Neurosurg Pediatr 2010; 6(6): 536-40.
[http://dx.doi.org/10.3171/2010.9.PEDS10267] [PMID: 21121727]

[12] Doddamani R, Kota R, Ahemad N, Chandra PS, Tripathi M. Minimally invasive hemispherotomy for refractory epilepsy in infants and young adults'. J Neurointerv Surg 2023; 15(9): 933-4.
[http://dx.doi.org/10.1136/jnis-2023-020076] [PMID: 36639232]

[13] Chandra PS, Doddamani RS, Samala R, *et al.* Endoscopic Hemispherotomy for Nonatrophic Rasmussen's Encephalopathy. Neurol India 2021; 69(4): 837-41.
[http://dx.doi.org/10.4103/0028-3886.325379] [PMID: 34507398]

[14] Chandra PS, Kurwale N, Garg A, Dwivedi R, Malviya SV, Tripathi M. Endoscopy-assisted interhemispheric transcallosal hemispherotomy: preliminary description of a novel technique. Neurosurgery 2015; 76(4): 485-95.
[http://dx.doi.org/10.1227/NEU.0000000000000675] [PMID: 25710106]

[15] Sood S, Marupudi NI, Asano E, Haridas A, Ham SD. Endoscopic corpus callosotomy and hemispherotomy. J Neurosurg Pediatr 2015; 16(6): 681-6.
[http://dx.doi.org/10.3171/2015.5.PEDS1531] [PMID: 26407094]

[16] Kotagal P, Lüders HO. Recent advances in childhood epilepsy. Brain Dev 1994; 16(1): 1-15.
[http://dx.doi.org/10.1016/0387-7604(94)90106-6] [PMID: 8059922]

[17] Villemure J, Rasmussen T. Functional hemispherectomy in children. Neuropediatrics 1993; 24(1): 53-5.
[http://dx.doi.org/10.1055/s-2008-1071514] [PMID: 8474613]

[18] Tinuper P, Andermann F, Villemure JG, Rasmussen TB, Quesney LF. Functional hemispherectomy for treatment of epilepsy associated with hemiplegia: Rationale, indications, results, and comparison with callosotomy. Ann Neurol 1988; 24(1): 27-34.
[http://dx.doi.org/10.1002/ana.410240107] [PMID: 3137858]

[19] Villemure JG. Anatomical to functional hemispherectomy from Krynauw to Rasmussen. Epilepsy Res Suppl 1992; 5: 209-15.
[PMID: 1418452]

[20] Rasmussen T, Villemure JG. Cerebral hemispherectomy for seizures with hemiplegia. Cleve Clin J Med 1989; 56 (Suppl.): S-62-8.

[http://dx.doi.org/10.3949/ccjm.56.s1.62] [PMID: 2655991]

[21] Bahuleyan B, Robinson S, Nair AR, Sivanandapanicker JL, Cohen AR. Anatomic hemispherectomy: historical perspective. World Neurosurg 2013; 80(3-4): 396-8.
[http://dx.doi.org/10.1016/j.wneu.2012.03.020] [PMID: 22480976]

[22] Villemure JG, Meagher-Villemure K, Montes JL, Farmer JP, Broggi G. Disconnective hemispherectomy for hemispheric dysplasia. Epileptic Disord 2003; 5(S2) (Suppl. 2): S125-30.
[http://dx.doi.org/10.1684/j.1950-6945.2003.tb00041.x] [PMID: 14617431]

[23] Villemure JG, Daniel RT. Peri-insular hemispherotomy in paediatric epilepsy. Childs Nerv Syst 2006; 22(8): 967-81.
[http://dx.doi.org/10.1007/s00381-006-0134-3] [PMID: 16804712]

[24] Nagel J, Elbabaa S, Hadar E, Bingaman W, Luders H. Hemispherectomy techniques Text Book of Epilepsy Surgery London. UK: Informa Healthcare 2008; pp. 1162-72.

[25] Delalande O, Dorfmüller G. [Parasagittal vertical hemispherotomy: surgical procedure]. Neurochirurgie 2008; 54(3): 353-7.
[http://dx.doi.org/10.1016/j.neuchi.2008.02.024] [PMID: 18433805]

[26] Wen HT, Rhoton AL Jr, Marino R Jr. Anatomical landmarks for hemispherotomy and their clinical application. J Neurosurg 2004; 101(5): 747-55.
[http://dx.doi.org/10.3171/jns.2004.101.5.0747] [PMID: 15540911]

[27] Delalande O, Bulteau C, Dellatolas G, *et al.* Vertical parasagittal hemispherotomy: surgical procedures and clinical long-term outcomes in a population of 83 children. Neurosurgery 2007; 60(2) (Suppl. 1): ONS19-32. [discussion ONS.].
[PMID: 17297362]

[28] Uda T, Tamrakar S, Tsuyuguchi N, *et al.* Anatomic Understanding of Vertical Hemispherotomy With Cadaveric Brains and Intraoperative Photographs. Oper Neurosurg (Hagerstown) 2016; 12(4): 374-82.
[http://dx.doi.org/10.1227/NEU.0000000000001272] [PMID: 29506282]

[29] Hinojosa J, Gil-Robles S, Pascual B. Clinical considerations and surgical approaches for low-grade gliomas in deep hemispheric locations: insular lesions. Childs Nerv Syst 2016; 32(10): 1875-93.
[http://dx.doi.org/10.1007/s00381-016-3183-2] [PMID: 27659830]

[30] Kucukyuruk B, Yagmurlu K, Tanriover N, Uzan M, Rhoton AL Jr. Microsurgical anatomy of the white matter tracts in hemispherotomy. Neurosurgery 2014; 10 (Suppl. 2): 305-24.
[PMID: 24448186]

[31] Gonçalves-Ferreira A, Campos AR, Herculano-Carvalho M, *et al.* Amygdalohippocampotomy: surgical technique and clinical results. J Neurosurg 2013; 118(5): 1107-13.
[http://dx.doi.org/10.3171/2013.1.JNS12727] [PMID: 23432145]

[32] Cook SW, Nguyen ST, Hu B, Yudovin S, Shields WD, Vinters HV, *et al.* Cerebral hemispherectomy in pediatric patients with epilepsy: comparison of three techniques by pathological substrate in 115 patients. J Neurosurg 2004; 100(2 Suppl Pediatrics): 125-41.

[33] Kwan A, Ng WH, Otsubo H, Ochi A, Snead OC 3rd, Tamber MS, *et al.* Hemispherectomy for the control of intractable epilepsy in childhood: comparison of 2 surgical techniques in a single institution. Neurosurgery 2010; 67(2 Suppl Operative): 429-36.
[http://dx.doi.org/10.1227/NEU.0b013e3181f743dc]

[34] Kiehna EN, Widjaja E, Holowka S, *et al.* Utility of diffusion tensor imaging studies linked to neuronavigation and other modalities in repeat hemispherotomy for intractable epilepsy. J Neurosurg Pediatr 2016; 17(4): 483-90.
[http://dx.doi.org/10.3171/2015.7.PEDS15101] [PMID: 26651159]

CHAPTER 8

Endoscopic Treatment for Early Correction of Craniosynostosis in Children

Leonardo Domínguez[1,2,*], Claudio Rivas-Palacios[1,3], Mario M. Barbosa[4], María Andrea Escobar[5,6], Elvira Puello F.[1,7] and Ezequiel García-Ballestas[1,3,8]

[1] *Department of Pediatric Neurosurgery. Napoleon Franco Pareja Children's Hospital (Child's House), Cartagena, Colombia*

[2] *Department of Neurosurgery, University of Cartagena, Cartagena, Colombia*

[3] *Center of Biomedical Research (CIB), Faculty of Medicine, University of Cartagena, Cartagena, Colombia*

[4] *Trauma and Emergency Epidemiology Research Group, University of Valle, Cali, Colombia*

[5] *Faculty of Medicine, Rafael Nuñez University, Cartagena, Colombia*

[6] *Department of Arts and Humanities, International University of Valencia, Valencia, Spain*

[7] *Faculty of Medicine, University El Sinu, Cartagena, Colombia*

[8] *Latinamerican Council of Neurocritical Care (CLaNI), Bogota, Colombia*

Abstract: Initial treatments for craniosynostosis involved strip craniectomies, but due to unsatisfactory results in advanced stages, extensive cranial remodeling was introduced, despite its risks and prolonged hospital stays. Over the last 30 years, strip craniectomies have seen a revival, primarily due to the incorporation of minimally invasive endoscopic-assisted surgeries (EAS) as pioneered by Jiménez and Barone. EAS has shown marked advantages over older surgical methods, including shorter surgical times, reduced bleeding, and fewer hospitalization requirements, all while achieving comparable results in cranial deformity corrections. The most influential factor in perioperative morbidity is surgical time. EAS has emerged as a promising, effective treatment for craniosynostosis, suggesting its wider adoption in neurosurgical settings. Considering the relationship between age, surgical time, and blood loss, EAS may be suitably extended to children aged 6-12 months.

Keywords: Craniosynostosis, Endoscopic-assisted surgeries, Strip craniectomies.

---

* **Corresponding autor Leonardo Domínguez:** Department of Pediatric Neurosurgery. Napoleon Franco Pareja Children's Hospital (Child's House), Cartagena, Colombia and Department of Neurosurgery, University of Cartagena, Cartagena, Colombia; E-mail: ledomi@yahoo.com

INTRODUCTION

Craniosynostosis represents a prevalent congenital craniofacial anomaly, stemming from the premature ossification and fusion of one or more cranial sutures [1, 2]. The ailment's classification spectrum ranges based on the suture involvement, delineating into simple or complex subtypes, and further categorized as primary or secondary forms [3]. Within the realm of primary craniosynostosis, distinctions arise between syndromic and non-syndromic variants, with the non-syndromic form being predominant [2 - 5]. Non-syndromic manifestations frequently include scaphocephaly, trigonocephaly, and anterior plagiocephaly presentations [2 - 6]. For their part, syndromic craniosynostosis commonly aligns with conditions such as Crouzon, Appert, Muenke, and Pfeiffer syndromes [3, 7 - 9]. This anomaly can result in a myriad of complications, encompassing craniofacial anomalies, sensory deficits, escalated intracranial pressure, and profound neurocognitive repercussions [2, 3, 9].

Historically, surgical interventions targeting craniosynostosis have evolved. Strip craniectomies once was the primary treatment, however, suboptimal outcomes precipitated their decline until a resurgence in the 1940s, emphasizing prophylactic and early interventions [10, 11]. Subsequent methodologies embraced expansive cranial reconstruction, albeit fraught with challenges such as elongated operative durations and significant hemorrhagic episodes [12 - 14]. A paradigm shift was observed in the 1990s with the advent of simplified endoscopic suturectomy, heralded as a novel approach [15]. This chapter describes the endoscopic-assisted surgery (EAS) juxtaposed against traditional open surgical methodologies in pediatric patients aged below 6 months. A synthesis of perioperative and reconstructive insights, derived from contemporary literature and bolstered by a rich 26-year institutional experience, will also be presented [16].

Open Surgical Technique

For all corrective interventions utilizing the Open Surgical Technique (OS), a standard procedural sequence is adhered to:

- **Incisions**: Ensuring the pericranium remains intact, strategic skin incisions are made. Notably, subperiosteal dissections are avoided.
- **Subgaleal Dissection**: A comprehensive subgaleal dissection is executed, interconnecting the separate incisions.
- **Dura Mater Dissection**: Utilizing Freer's dissector, a separation of the dura mater and the subjacent dural sinuses from the amalgamated sagittal suture is accomplished.

Condition-Specific Surgical Protocols:

Scaphocephaly (≤ 3 months):

- *Positioning*: The patient is oriented supinely, maintaining head neutrality and an inflected neck.
- *Incision*: A parasagittal "C" incision, originating from the coronal region and terminating at the lambda, is affected.
- *Sagittal Synostectomy*: A sagittal synostectomy spanning 4-5 cm is conducted.

Scaphocephaly (> 3 – 6 months):

- *Positioning*: The patient is positioned supinely in a semi-Fowler stance, ensuring head neutrality.
- *Incision*: A sinuous incision is made equidistant between the bregma and lambda, extending from one ear to the other (Fig. **1A**).
- *Burr Holes & Craniectomy*: Utilizing a craniotome, 4 trepanation portals are established – two retro bregmatic and two prelimbic, situated 2 cm away from the bilateral median. Following this, a 4-5 cm sagittal synostectomy and a subsequent craniectomy (measuring 1-2 cm) are performed.

Trigonocephaly:

- *Positioning*: With the head adjusted to a zero-degree inclination, the patient is positioned supinely.
- *Incision & Craniectomy*: A sinuous incision stretching between the ears is made, coinciding with the coronal territory (Fig. **1C**). A craniotome creates a burr hole over the stenotic metopic suture, which is elongated towards the anterior fontanelle. A metopic synostectomy of dimensions 2 cm x 3-4 cm is executed.

Anterior Plagiocephaly:

- *Positioning*: Patients are oriented supinely with their heads directed to the plagiocephaly's opposite side, revealing the affected frontotemporal region.
- *Incision & Craniectomy*: A coronal incision on the plagiocephalic side is rendered. Thereafter, a pair of trephination apertures are created, followed by a 2 cm wide retro coronal craniectomy.

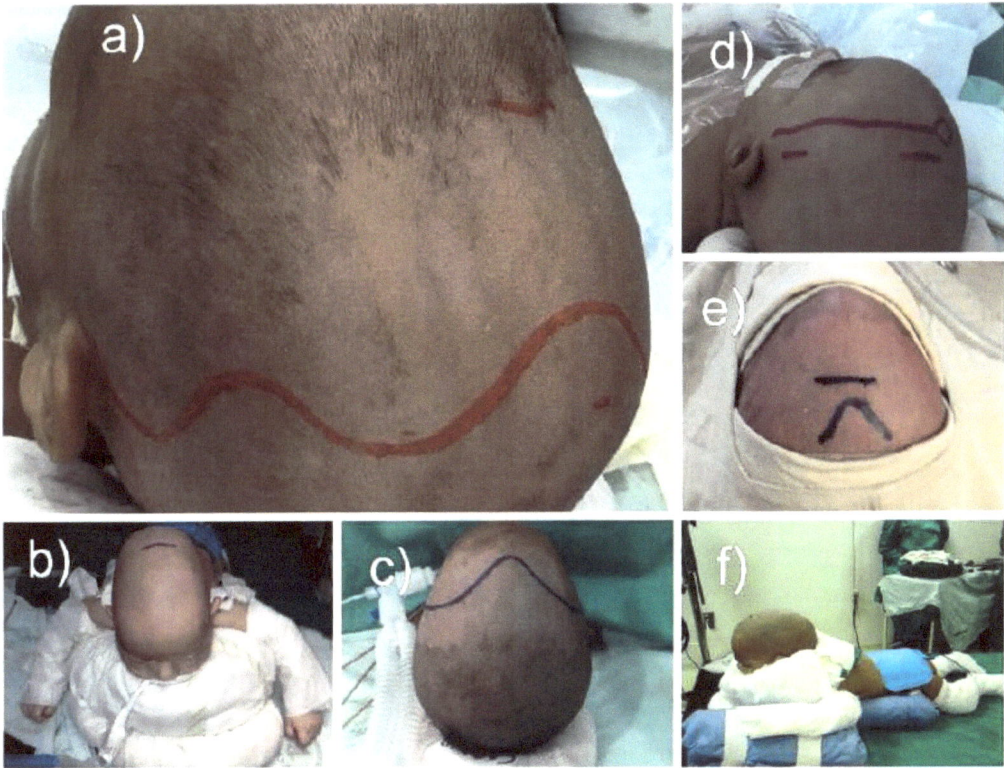

Fig. (1). Dissection strategies, anatomical orientations, and postoperative nuances in both OS and EAS are as follows: a) A serpentine incision is made, traversing from one auditory region to the other, equidistant from the bregma and lambda during the OS scaphocephaly procedure. b) In the context of EAS scaphocephaly, a pair of dermal incisions are made: one being retro coronal (retro bregmatic) and the other lambdoidal; each spanning approximately 3-4 cm. c) For OS trigonocephaly and anterior plagiocephaly, a sinuous incision is produced between the auditory regions, aligned with the coronal plane. d) With EAS anterior plagiocephaly, two linear incisions of 2 cm are made: one retro coronal, situated laterally to the anterior fontanelle, and its counterpart being retro coronal temporal, in congruence with the ossified suture. e) A horizontal epidermal incision, approximately 2-3 cm in length, is produced posterior to the hairline but anterior to the fontanelle during trigonocephaly interventions. f) For EAS scaphocephaly management, patients are positioned in a nuanced sphinx orientation. b) Strategic positioning of spatulas: the former being subgaleal and the latter situated epidurally. c) A pair of epidermal incisions are made: one retro coronal (retro bregmatic) with its counterpart being lambdoidal. d) Detailed exposure of the retrocoronal incision. e-f) The neuroendoscope, accessing *via* the retrocoronal incision, is involved in the intricate sagittal synostectomy process. g) A comprehensive monoblock cystectomy extraction is executed. h) Bifurcated incision suture application.

Acrocephaly:

• This procedural approach mirrors the aforementioned plagiocephaly technique but is implemented bilaterally.

Endoscopically Assisted surgical Techniques

Utilizing the endoscopy-assisted surgical methodology as set forth by Jiménez and Barone [15], a defined set of instruments is required: a neuroendoscope equipped with 0 and 30-degree optics, coupled with the specialized Jiménez separator (subgaleal and epidural spatula). The principal procedural steps for endoscopy-assisted corrections are delineated as follows (refer to Figs. **1** & **2**):

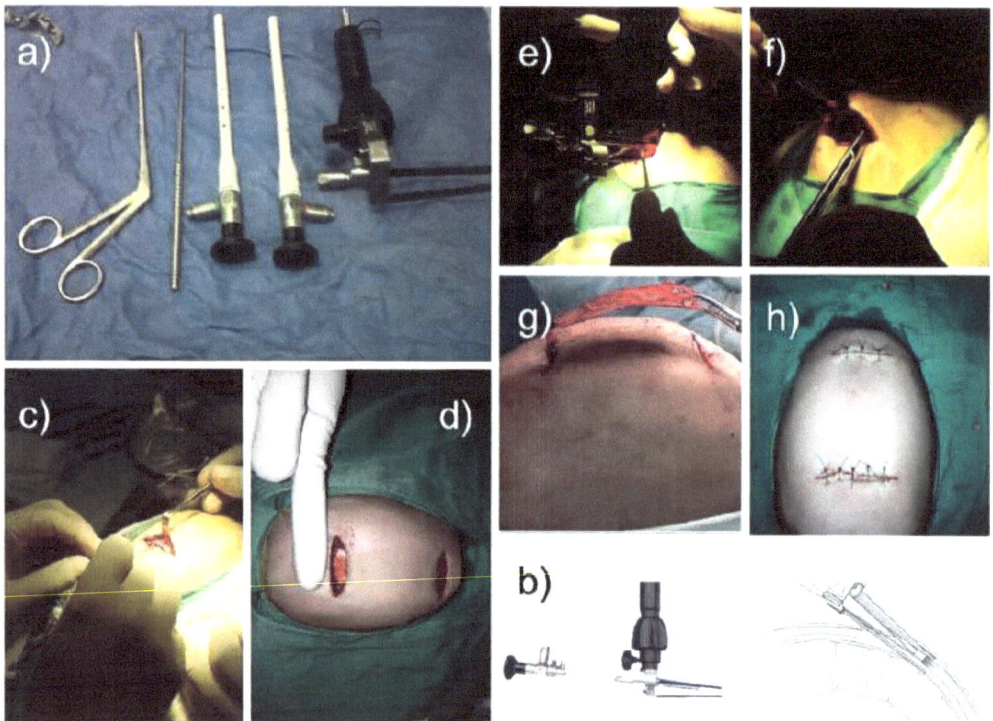

Fig. (2). Endoscopic management of sagittal synostosis entails: a) Utilization of a neuroendoscope equipped with dual optical configurations of 0 and 30 degrees, in conjunction with a Jiménez separator designed for both subgaleal and epidural interventions.

- Strategically placed skin incisions ensure the preservation of the pericranium, whilst circumventing subperiosteal dissection.
- The interstice between the two incisions is subjected to a comprehensive subgaleal dissection, employing a Freer dissector.
- With the aid of endoscopic magnification (a 30-degree lens for trigonocephaly cases, and a 0-degree lens for alternative synostoses), a meticulous dissection of the dura mater and the affiliated dural sinuses associated with the consolidated sagittal suture is achieved using the Freer dissector.

• Continuing under endoscopic guidance (30-degree lens for trigonocephaly and 0 degrees for other synostoses), both synostectomy and strip craniectomy are executed, employing Mayo scissors (refer to Fig. **3**).

Specific techniques are employed for different types of craniosynostosis:

For each cranial deformity, a specific protocol is utilized, distinguished by anatomical placements, incisional strategies, and intervention techniques:

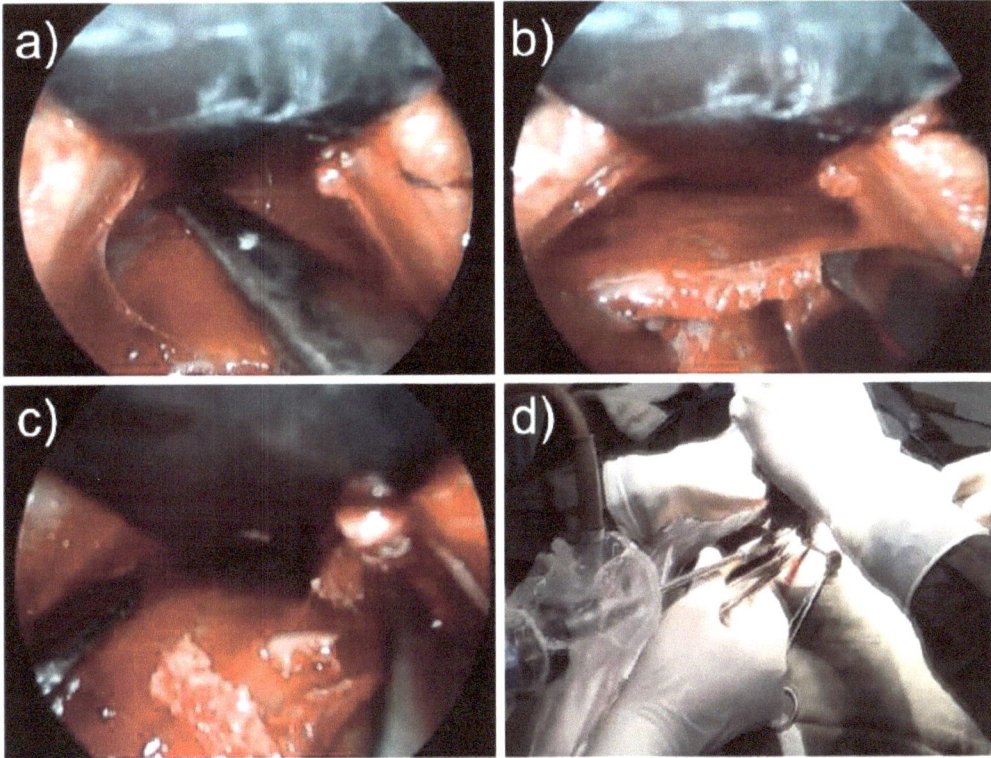

Fig. (3). Under 0-degree endoscopic visualization for sagittal synostosis correction: a) Utilizing Freer's dissector across the span between two dermal incisions, interventions on the subgaleal region, dura mater, and the affiliated dural sinuses of the conjoined sagittal suture are executed; b) A sagittal cystectomy of approximately 4-5 cm in width is undertaken using Mayo scissors, culminating at the intersection with retrocoronal and prelimbic craniotomies; c) Comprehensive removal of the monoblock cystectomy is achieved; meticulous scrutiny of the entirety of the dura mater is conducted to detect any inadvertent ruptures; d) Dual surgical approach: Surgeon 1, positioned adjacently to the patient and oriented at zero degrees, assumes responsibility for craniotomies and associated dissections. Conversely, Surgeon 2, stationed at an angle between 15-30 degrees relative to the patient, manages the neuroendoscope.

• **Scaphocephaly**: The patient is placed into a prone or a nuanced sphinx position, as illustrated in reference [15] (See Fig. **1B & F**). Two precision skin incisions are executed: a retro coronal (retro bregmatic) and a lambdoid, spanning 3-4 cm (Refer to Fig. **1B**). Utilizing a craniotome, four burr holes are created: a bilateral pair retro bregmatic and another lambdoid; each stationed 2 cm off the midline. The trepanation orifices are extended anteriorly to the fontanelle and the lambdoid suture, employing Gouge forceps. Subsequent procedures entail a retro coronal band craniectomy of 4-5 cm in length, a pre-lambdoid band of the same length, and a sagittal synostectomy of 4-5 cm in width, culminating in the extraction of the monoblock synostectomy.

• **Trigonocephaly**: With the patient in supine orientation, the cranium is maintained at a zero-degree tilt. A transverse incision of approximately 2-3 cm is made behind the hairline proximal to the anterior fontanelle (Fig. **1E**). Directly above the constricted metopic suture, a craniotome is used to produce a burr hole. The burr aperture is extended longitudinally to the anterior fontanelle *via* gouge forceps. A metopic synostectomy, measuring 2 cm in width and 3-4 cm in length, is pursued using the craniotome. The osteotomy, facilitated by gouge forceps, advances proximate to the nasofrontal suture.

• **Anterior Plagiocephaly**: The patient is supine, cranium rotated to juxtapose the non-affected plagiocephaly side, thus revealing the frontotemporal region under duress. Twin longitudinal incisions of 2 cm are made: one retro coronal, adjacent to the anterior fontanelle, and a counterpart retro coronal temporal, aligned with the ossified suture (Fig. **1D**). Employing a craniotome, a pair of trephination portals are cut: one laterally juxtaposed to the anterior fontanelle on the stenosed coronal suture, and its companion pterional. The culmination is a retro coronal strip craniectomy, 2 cm wide, anchored at the pterion.

• **Acrocephaly**: This process adheres closely to the anterior plagiocephaly procedure, but manifests bilaterally.

Craniometric Assessments, Cranial Defect Estimation, and Follow-up

During the preoperative evaluation, precise craniometric evaluations are imperative for each patient. For diagnosing scaphocephaly and acrocephaly, the cranial index (CI) is employed, while the cranial asymmetry index (CAI) becomes pertinent for anterior plagiocephaly presentations. In the context of trigonocephaly, the ratio juxtaposing bicoronal and biparietal distances (BCD/BPD) is computed. With these metrics established, the cranial deficit percentage of every patient is ascertained in alignment with their specific craniometric data. Benchmark values are set at CI $\geq$ 74% for scaphocephaly, $\leq$ 84% for acrocephaly, CAI $\leq$ 3.5, and a BCD/BPD value of 1.21 – in excess of which is considered aberrant. Postoperative assessments are scheduled at intervals of one month, three months, and subsequently, a year.

Perioperative Outcomes

With the advent of craniosynostosis rectification *via* the Endoscopic-Assisted Surgery (EAS) methodology, there has been an escalating inclination towards its adoption. Comparative studies underscore superior perioperative outcomes with EAS *vis-à-vis* the Open Surgical (OS) approach. EAS boasts demonstrable advantages, including diminished Estimated Blood Loss (EBL), decreased transfusion requisites, reduced operative durations, abbreviated hospitalization periods, and lesser Intensive Care Unit (ICU) deployment relative to OS. Subsequently, an analytical juxtaposition delineating contrasts between EAS and OS modalities will be provided.

Surgical Time

Numerous reports highlight a diminished operative duration for Endoscopic-Assisted Surgery (EAS) relative to the Open Surgical (OS) modality [15, 17, 18, 20, 28 - 36]. A comprehensive multicenter analysis involving 1,382 pediatric patients, aged below 12 months, yielded an average surgical time of 70 minutes for EAS versus 115 minutes for OS [21]. In our own institution, there was a marked decrement in surgical duration for those receiving EAS as opposed to OS interventions [16], as illustrated in Table **1** and Fig. (**4C**). The expedited techniques integral to EAS, typified by succinct skin incisions, monolithic synostectomies, and strip craniectomies, are pivotal to its abbreviated procedural span [15, 29, 37]. Intriguingly, age does not appear to be a determinant affecting operative duration [29]. Conversely, the specific suture in question can affect surgical times [20]. It is important to emphasize that operative duration has been identified as the foremost risk factor for intraoperative hemorrhage during craniosynostosis rectification, as corroborated by various scholars [16, 38 - 40].

Table 1. Patient demographic data and perioperative results.

Characteristics	Overall (N=74)	Open (N=24)	Endoscopic (N=50)	p-value
Age (months)	4.75 (3.00, 5.00)	5.00 (4.00, 5.25)	4.00 (3.00, 5.00)	0.013
Gender:	-	-	-	0.8
Female	29 (39%)	10 (42%)	19 (38%)	-
Male	45 (61%)	14 (58%)	31 (62%)	-
Surgical time (min)	45 (35, 105)	116 (105, 128)	35 (30, 45)	<0.001
EBL (ml)	38 (30, 131)	165 (146, 181)	32 (28, 38)	<0.001
Bleeding percentage of EBV	9 (6, 25)	29 (25, 32)	6 (5, 9)	<0.001
Transfusion of blood products	23 (31%)	19 (79%)	4 (8.0%)	<0.001
Use of TXA	22 (30%)	20 (83%)	2 (4.0%)	<0.001

(Table 1) cont.....

Characteristics	Overall (N=74)	Open (N=24)	Endoscopic (N=50)	p-value
Transfusion in patients with TXA	22 (95.6%)	19 (95%)	2 (100%)	0.9
Complications (Dural Tear, Surgical Site Infection)				
infection)	0	0	0	-
Hospital stay (days)	1 (1, 2)	4 (3, 4)	1 (1, 1)	<0.001
ICU admission	8 (10.8%)	8 (33.33%)	0 (0%)	<0.001

Adapted from Dominguez *et al.* "Outcomes of endoscopic treatment for early correction of craniosynostosis in children: a 26-year single center experience." Journal of Neurosurgery: Pediatrics. 2023;1(aop):1-10.

Estimated Blood Loss (EBL)

Individuals subjected to EAS demonstrated markedly reduced EBL and proportional bleedings of EBV when juxtaposed against those managed *via* OS [15 - 18, 20, 28, 30 - 34], as depicted in Table **1** and Fig. (**4A**) & (**4B**). Noteworthy contributions from Jiménez and Barone [29], as well as Dalle Ore *et al.* [20], indicate an average EBL reduction to a mere 25 ml in EAS interventions. This decrement in EBL observed with EAS is associated with factors such as concise skin incisions, minimized osseous exposure, and the expedient adoption of strip craniectomies eschewing subperiosteal dissection, all compounded by a reduced surgical span [15, 17, 18, 20, 24, 28 - 36]. Intriguingly, a robust correlation exists between operative duration and EBL, implying that protracted surgical interventions promote an augmented EBL [16]. Such observations resonate with the wider academic consensus, which deems surgical time to be a predictor of elevated EBL during craniosynostosis remediation [38 - 40]. Although age's association with EBL is detectable yet devoid of linearity [16], Jiménez and Barone discerned an insensitivity of age *vis-à-vis* EBL amplitude [29]. It is important to underscore that the magnitude of EBL is invariably linked to the specific variant of synostosis under therapeutic consideration, given the unique pathophysiological nuances innate to different sutural types [19, 40].

Transfusion of Blood Products

Within our institutional experience, only 8% of EAS recipients necessitated transfusion of hematological products, a figure dramatically diminished compared to their OS counterparts [16] as delineated in Tables **1** and **2**. Diverse studies have reported transfusion requirements between 4% and 10% for EAS [20, 33, 47 - 50]. Notably, Mendonca *et al.* identified a complete absence of transfusions amidst a cohort of 17 EAS subjects [17]. In stark contrast, findings by Melin *et al.* [18], Honeycutt *et al.* [19], Dalle Ore *et al.* [20], and Thompson *et al.* [21] reported transfusion frequencies of 42%, 23%, 46.7%, and 26%, respectively. It merits emphasis that pediatric patients, beyond the age of four months and devoid of concurrent pathologies, can adeptly weather declines in hemoglobin concentrations to 7 g/dl, provided they retain normovolemia [22]. This physiological tenet may explain instances of zero transfusion propensities in EAS cohorts, especially when post-surgical hemoglobin thresholds hovered around 6 g/dl in patients with uncompromised hemodynamic levels [23]. Adjuvant modalities encompassing perioperative tranexamic acid (TXA), erythropoietin (EPO), and antecedent parenteral iron infusion have been tactically deployed to attenuate EBL and transfusion exigencies in craniosynostosis interventions [24 - 27]. A report from Children's Hospital of Richmond (CHoR) [26] described a regimen including antecedent recombinant EPO and iron provisioning, intraoperative autotransfusion, and the endorsement of hemoglobin concentrations sub-seven g/dl. Nonetheless, this series manifested a 56% transfusion requirement in patients within the regimen's ambit, without specification of the operative modality employed [26]. In our data set, a mere 4% of EAS beneficiaries were administered TXA, juxtaposed against a substantial 78% in the OS cohort. Yet, TXA's role in transfusion mitigation remained inconclusive for both groups (Table **1**). Remarkably, EAS robustly diminished the propensity for hematological product transfusion, with a staggering 99-fold decrement [16] (Table **2**). Corroboratively, a comprehensive meta-analysis encompassing seven inquiries (n = 1600) unequivocally underscored the attenuated transfusion prevalence in EAS recipients *vis-à-vis* OS (OR = 0.09, CI = 0.03-0.26, p < 0.001) [28].

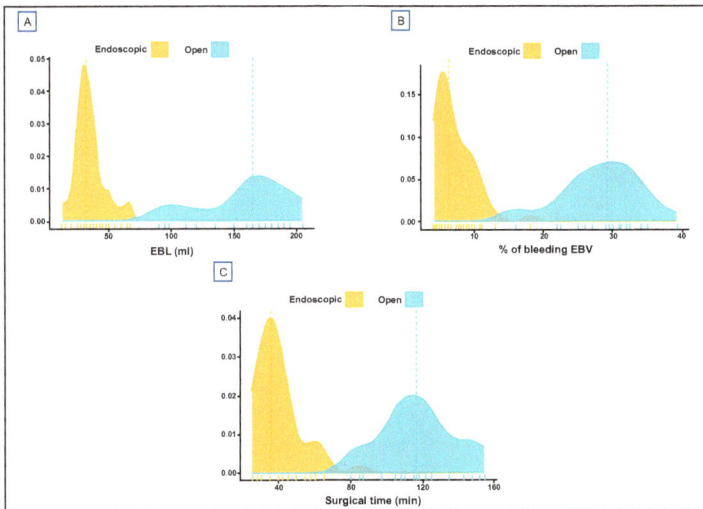

Fig. (4). Perioperative metrics encompassing estimated blood loss (EBL) (A), proportional deviation in effective blood volume (EBV) (B), and operative duration (C) are depicted. The vertical axis indicates quantified metrics juxtaposed against the horizontal axis variables. This illustration has been adapted from Dominguez *et al.*'s seminal work titled, "Endoscopic Interventions for Pediatric Craniosynostosis: A 26-Year Singular Institutional Review," as published in the Journal of Neurosurgery: Pediatrics, 2023;1(aop):110.

Table 2. Transfusion of blood products.

Age	Endoscopic Overall (N=23) Open (N=21) (N=4) OR	p-value
≤ 4 months: EBL > 10% EBV	12 8 4 0.18 (0.081 - 0.423)	<0.001
> 4 months: EBL > MEBL		

Adapted from Dominguez *et al.* "Outcomes of endoscopic treatment for early correction of center experience". Journal of Neurosurgery: Pediatrics. 2023;1(aop):1-10.

Postoperative Hospital Stay

Patients subjected to EAS typically necessitated only a single day of hospitalization, in contrast to the OS cohort which averaged a four-day duration [14, 16 - 18, 28 - 35]. Within our institutional records, the EAS group required zero intensive care unit (ICU) commitments, whereas a striking 33.33% of the OS group found themselves under ICU care [16], as depicted in Table **1**. This trend resonates with existing literature, wherein the OS cohort predominantly warranted intensive therapeutic oversight [17, 21, 31]. Riordan *et al.*, in their expansive analysis of 500 EAS participants, documented ICU requirements in a modest 3.2% fraction [36]. A multicentric assessment juxtaposing these surgical groups revealed a pervasive ICU admission trend for EAS candidates in a mere 40% (8 of 20) of the surveyed establishments. Conversely, the OS cohort experienced postoperative ICU admission in a substantial 83% (24 out of 29) of institutions [21]. While ICU incorporation post-OS for craniosynostosis emerges as a recurrent theme, it is imperative to recalibrate postoperative care, tailoring it to individual needs. Such a bespoke approach could lead to a marked curtailment in ICU admissions by consistently observing meticulously crafted admission paradigms [41, 42].

Surgery Cost

In our study, while a granular economic analysis was not conducted, the cumulative benefits of EAS – encompassing reduced surgical durations, minimized intraoperative pharmacological interventions, diminished transfusion necessities, shortened hospitalization periods, and a reduction in subsequent ICU admissions – imply a financially more prudent methodology as compared with OS. In a meticulous inquiry, Gerety *et al.* illuminated the pronounced financial disparity, determining that the fiscal obligation for OS was thrice its EAS counterpart ($35,280 vs. $13,147). Notably, this calculation remained consistent even when accounting for ancillary expenditures like spring extractions and cranial reconfigurations employing orthotic therapies [43]. A retrospective examination from St. Louis Children's Hospital located in Washington, D.C. indicated that the cost impositions for the OS cohort approximated $40,687, in sharp contrast to the $18,450 calculated for EAS [52, 53]. Subsequent research published by this establishment further corroborated these economic figures [34].

Cranial Index Correction

During the early stages of EAS adoption, a prevailing apprehension pertained to its aesthetic efficacy *vis-à-vis* OS. A compendium of research has documented similar cranial index (CI) improvements at 12, 24, and 48 months across both therapeutic modalities [34, 43 - 49]. A systematic review by Thwin *et al.* juxtaposed the average CI metamorphosis a year post-operatively, positing a slight advantage for OS over EAS in cases characterized by isolated sagittal suture synostosis. Nevertheless, as indicated across diverse studies, both interventions manifested enduring enhancements in cranial aberrations, with success rate percentages between 95% and 104% [50]. Upon retrospective analysis of our own institutional data encompassing acrocephaly and scaphocephaly cohorts, the OS subset exhibited a more pronounced CI rectification in the immediate postoperative month. However, subsequent observations at the 3- and 12-month milestones showcased negligible disparities (Table **3**) (Fig. **5**). An intriguing study by Al-Shaqsi *et al.*, wherein a continuum of follow-up imagery of a scaphocephalic patient was presented to 538 evaluators, indicated that the societal benchmark for an acceptable sagittal craniosynostosis rectification approximated 70% of the extant deformity [51]. Admittedly, within numerous clinical circles, helmet therapy has been lauded as an integral post-EAS craniosynostosis rectification tool. Yet, in our operational environment, these helmets remain scarce and financially prohibitive. Thus, contingent on this reality, helmet therapy was judiciously prescribed predominantly for coronal synostosis cases (encompassing both unilateral and bilateral presentations), given the intricate nature of their craniofacial irregularities [16] (Fig. **5**).

Table 3. Postoperative CI correction percentage

Follow-up	Overall (N=34)	Open (N=13)	Endocospic (N=21)	p-value
1 month	15.0 (14.00, 16.10)	16.9 (15.47, 18.22)	14.9 (13.83, 15.30)	<0.00 1
3 months	54.5 (52.1, 58.7)	56.5 (51.0, 60.8)	54.0 (52.4, 56.0)	0.4
12 months	97.3 (96.0, 100.6)	98.0 (96.8, 102.0)	97.0 (96.0, 99.0)	0.3

Adapted from Dominguez *et al.* "Outcomes of endoscopic treatment for early correction of craniosynostosis in children: a 26-year single center experience." Journal of Neurosurgery: Pediatrics. 2023;1(aop):1-10.

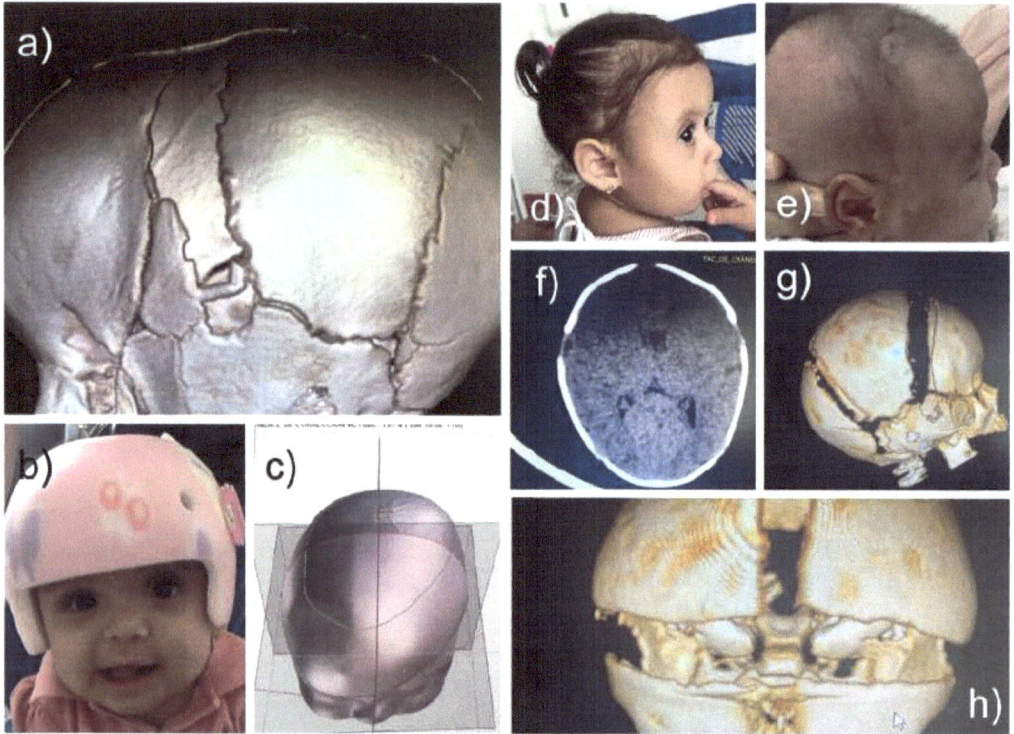

Fig. (5). Postoperative results of EAS-mediated cranial rectification are illustrated as follows: a) Tridimensional cranial tomography subsequent to a unilateral coronal synostectomy; b & c) Anterior plagiocephaly necessitating orthotic helmet intervention; d) Twelve-month follow-up depicts cranial malformation remediation exceeding 80%; e - g) Tomographic imaging coupled with tridimensional post-surgical reconstructions exemplifying acrocephalia amelioration; h) A trimestrial post-surgical appraisal post acrocephalia intervention, highlighting cranial anomaly correction surpassing 50%.

Optimal Correction Time

Multiple scholarly investigations corroborate that the prime window for early EAS intervention falls within the initial three months of life [17, 46, 54]. During this period, the cranium retains its malleability, evidenced by the frontal and parietal bone thickness remaining under 2 mm [55, 56], thereby simplifying strip craniectomies. Within our clinical setting, patients typically presented for EAS at an average age of four months, with ages spanning from 15 days up to six months. This chronological boundary was set in light of the observed bone thickness progression in frontal and parietal regions which, by half a year, approximates a range of 2.5-3 mm [55, 56]. It should be noted that during the first six months, there is an accentuated cranial growth rate paired with significant bony pliancy. This scenario enables the encephalic mass to act as an inherent distractor, furthering cranial enlargement [17]. While certain facilities offer minimally invasive craniosynostosis interventions for the demographic aged between 6 to 11 months [29, 37], our institution adheres to a stringent criterion, limiting EAS to those below six months of age. Intriguingly, emerging research contends that for infants below a year old with sagittal synostosis, age does not definitively influence cranial microanatomy or its suppleness [55]. Given that, by one year of age, frontal and parietal bone densities typically attain a range of 3-4 mm [56], an argument could be made in favor of considering EAS up until this age milestone.

DISCUSSION

Initially, craniosynostosis management predominantly employed strip craniectomies [10, 11]. Yet, suboptimal outcomes in advanced disease stages catalyzed the development of alternative methodologies such as extensive cranial remodeling [13, 14]. Despite its efficacy, this modality presented challenges, including notable intraoperative hemorrhage, transfusion requisites, potential dural lacerations, extended surgical periods, and prolonged inpatient periods. Over recent decades, strip craniectomies have re-emerged in craniosynostosis therapeutic paradigms. This renewed interest is largely attributed to the proliferated adoption of minimally invasive strategies augmented by endoscopic guidance, as pioneeringly illustrated by Jiménez and Barone [15, 29]. EAS, when deployed early for craniosynostosis, exhibits pronounced advantages, notably diminished EBL, transfusion needs, operative durations, hospitalization, and ICU interventions *vis-à-vis* OS. Moreover, the comparative analysis indicates congruent cranial deformity rectification outcomes across both modalities. Of all the parameters, operative duration most significantly impacts perioperative morbidity.

In light of these observations, EAS emerges as a judicious and potent therapeutic avenue for craniosynostosis. We ardently advocate for its broader incorporation within eligible neurosurgical establishments. Further, given the correlative nuances between age, operative duration, EBL, and the documented cranial bone metrics in the 6–12-month cohort, there exists a compelling rationale to contemplate EAS extension within this age spectrum.

CONCLUSION

The evolution of craniosynostosis management has been marked by a progression from initial reliance on strip craniectomies through a phase of alternative methods due to suboptimal outcomes, culminating in the recent revival of strip craniectomies – enhanced by minimally invasive and endoscopic techniques. As spearheaded by Jiménez and Barone [15, 29], these modern methodologies, particularly the early application of EAS, offer significant improvements in treatment outcomes, surgical efficiency, and patient recovery. Notably, despite the differences in surgical techniques, both traditional and contemporary approaches have achieved comparable results in cranial deformity corrections. However, it is imperative to underscore the critical role that operative duration plays in influencing perioperative outcomes. The emergent evidence strongly posits EAS as a superior, efficient, and viable treatment modality for craniosynostosis. Encouraging its adoption in neurosurgical centers equipped with the necessary expertise appears prudent. Additionally, the interplay between age, surgical time, and cranial metrics in infants aged 6-12 months presents a strong case for broadening the applicability of EAS to encompass this age bracket.

REFERENCES

[1]   Xue AS, Buchanan EP, Hollier LH Jr. Update in management of craniosynostosis. Plast Reconstr Surg 2022; 149(6): 1209e-23e.
[http://dx.doi.org/10.1097/PRS.0000000000009046] [PMID: 35613293]

[2]   Chico Ponce de León F. Craneoestenosis. I. Bases biológicas y análisis de las craneoestenosis no sindromáticas. Bol Méd Hosp Infant México 2011; 68(5): 333-48.

[3]   Syndromic craniosynostosis: complexities of clinical care. Molecular syndromology 2019; 10(1-2): 83-97.

[4]   Persing JA. MOC-PS(SM) CME article: management considerations in the treatment of craniosynostosis. Plast Reconstr Surg 2008; 121(4) (Suppl.): 1-11.
[http://dx.doi.org/10.1097/01.prs.0000305929.40363.bf] [PMID: 18379381]

[5]   Dempsey RF, Monson LA, Maricevich RS, *et al.* Nonsyndromic Craniosynostosis. Clin Plast Surg 2019; 46(2): 123-39.
[http://dx.doi.org/10.1016/j.cps.2018.11.001] [PMID: 30851746]

[6]   Thompson D. Craniosynostosis-pathophysiology, clinical presentation, and investigation. Pediatr Neurosurg 1999; 275-90.

[7]   Otto AW. Lehrbuch der pathologischen Anatomie des Menschen und der Thiere: August Rücker 1830.

[8]   Virchow R. Uber den Cretinismus, samentlich in Franken, und uber pathologische schadelformen. Verh Phys Med Ges Wurz 1851; 2: 230-70.

[9]   Stanton E, Urata M, Chen JF, Chai Y. The clinical manifestations, molecular mechanisms and treatment of craniosynostosis. Dis Model Mech 2022; 15(4)dmm049390
[http://dx.doi.org/10.1242/dmm.049390] [PMID: 35451466]

[10]   Lane LC. Pioneer craniectomy for relief of mental imbecility due to premature sutural closure and microcephalus. JAMA 1892; XVIII(2): 49-50.
[http://dx.doi.org/10.1001/jama.1892.02411060019001f]

[11]   Lannelongue M. De la craniectomie dans la microcephalie. CR Acad Sci 1890; 110: 1382-5.

[12]   Lee JS, Yu JW. Craniosynostosis surgery The History of Maxillofacial Surgery: An Evidence-Based Journey. Springer 2022; pp. 367-90.
[http://dx.doi.org/10.1007/978-3-030-89563-1_20]

[13]   Mehta VA, Bettegowda C, Jallo GI, Ahn ES. The evolution of surgical management for craniosynostosis. Neurosurg Focus 2010; 29(6)E5
[http://dx.doi.org/10.3171/2010.9.FOCUS10204] [PMID: 21121719]

[14]   Tessier P. The definitive plastic surgical treatment of the severe facial deformities of craniofacial dysostosis. Crouzon's and Apert's diseases. Plast Reconstr Surg 1971; 48(5): 419-42.
[http://dx.doi.org/10.1097/00006534-197111000-00002] [PMID: 4942075]

[15]   Jimenez DF, Barone CM. Endoscopic craniectomy for early surgical correction of sagittal

craniosynostosis. J Neurosurg 1998; 88(1): 77-81.
[http://dx.doi.org/10.3171/jns.1998.88.1.0077] [PMID: 9420076]

[16]　Domínguez L, Rivas-Palacios C, Barbosa MM, Escobar MA, Florez EP, García-Ballestas E. Outcomes of endoscopic treatment for early correction of craniosynostosis in children: a 26-year single-center experience. Journal of Neurosurgery: Pediatrics 2023; 1(aop): 1-10.

[17]　Mendonca DA, Gopal S, Gujjalanavar R, Deraje V. HR S, Ramamurthy V. Endoscopic versus open cranial reconstruction surgery for anterior craniosynostosis: experience from South-East Asia. FACE 2020; 1(2): 105-13.
[http://dx.doi.org/10.1177/2732501620973034]

[18]　Melin AA, Moffitt J, Hopkins DC, *et al.* Is less actually more? An evaluation of surgical outcomes between endoscopic suturectomy and open cranial vault remodeling for craniosynostosis. J Craniofac Surg 2020; 31(4): 924-6.
[http://dx.doi.org/10.1097/SCS.0000000000006152] [PMID: 32049919]

[19]　Honeycutt JH, Ed. Endoscopic-assisted craniosynostosis surgery Seminars in plastic surgery. Thieme Medical Publishers 2014.

[20]　Dalle Ore CL, Dilip M, Brandel MG, *et al.* Endoscopic surgery for nonsyndromic craniosynostosis: a 16-year single-center experience. J Neurosurg Pediatr 2018; 22(4): 335-43.
[http://dx.doi.org/10.3171/2018.2.PEDS17364] [PMID: 29979128]

[21]　Thompson DR, Zurakowski D, Haberkern CM, *et al.* Endoscopic versus open repair for craniosynostosis in infants using propensity score matching to compare outcomes: a multicenter study from the Pediatric Craniofacial Collaborative Group. Anesth Analg 2018; 126(3): 968-75.
[http://dx.doi.org/10.1213/ANE.0000000000002454] [PMID: 28922233]

[22]　Zuluaga Giraldo M. Manejo del sangrado perioperatorio en niños. Revisión paso a paso. Revista Colombiana de Anestesiología 2013; 41(1): 50-6.
[http://dx.doi.org/10.1016/j.rca.2012.07.011]

[23]　Steinbok P, Heran N, Hicdonmez T, Cochrane DD, Price A. Minimizing blood transfusions in the surgical correction of coronal and metopic craniosynostosis. Childs Nerv Syst 2004; 20(7): 445-52.
[http://dx.doi.org/10.1007/s00381-004-0972-9] [PMID: 15168053]

[24]　Bonfield CM, Sharma J, Cochrane DD, Singhal A, Steinbok P. Minimizing blood transfusions in the surgical correction of craniosynostosis: a 10-year single-center experience. Childs Nerv Syst 2016; 32(1): 143-51.
[http://dx.doi.org/10.1007/s00381-015-2900-6] [PMID: 26351073]

[25]　Knackstedt R, Patel N. Enhanced recovery protocol after fronto-orbital advancement reduces transfusions, narcotic usage, and length of stay. Plast Reconstr Surg Glob Open 2020; 8(10)e3205
[http://dx.doi.org/10.1097/GOX.0000000000003205] [PMID: 33173704]

[26]　Vega RA, Lyon C, Kierce JF, Tye GW, Ritter AM, Rhodes JL. Minimizing transfusion requirements for children undergoing craniosynostosis repair: the CHoR protocol. J Neurosurg Pediatr 2014; 14(2): 190-5.
[http://dx.doi.org/10.3171/2014.4.PEDS13449] [PMID: 24877603]

[27]　Wei Y, Zhang Y, Jin T, Wang H, Li J, Zhang D. Effects of Tranexamic Acid on Bleeding in Pediatric Surgeries: A Systematic Review and Meta-Analysis. Front Surg 2021; 8759937
[http://dx.doi.org/10.3389/fsurg.2021.759937] [PMID: 34722626]

[28]　Goyal A, Lu VM, Yolcu YU, Elminawy M, Daniels DJ. Endoscopic versus open approach in craniosynostosis repair: a systematic review and meta-analysis of perioperative outcomes. Childs Nerv Syst 2018; 34(9): 1627-37.
[http://dx.doi.org/10.1007/s00381-018-3852-4] [PMID: 29961085]

[29]　Jimenez DF, McGinity MJ, Barone CM. Endoscopy-assisted early correction of single-suture metopic craniosynostosis: a 19-year experience. J Neurosurg Pediatr 2019; 23(1): 61-74.

[http://dx.doi.org/10.3171/2018.6.PEDS1749] [PMID: 30265229]

[30]   Han RH, Nguyen DC, Bruck BS, *et al.* Characterization of complications associated with open and endoscopic craniosynostosis surgery at a single institution. J Neurosurg Pediatr 2016; 17(3): 361-70. [http://dx.doi.org/10.3171/2015.7.PEDS15187] [PMID: 26588461]

[31]   Fassl V, Ellermann L, Reichelt G, *et al.* Endoscopic treatment of sagittal suture synostosis — a critical analysis of current management strategies. Neurosurg Rev 2022; 45(4): 2533-46. [http://dx.doi.org/10.1007/s10143-022-01762-y] [PMID: 35384543]

[32]   Proctor MR. Endoscopic cranial suture release for the treatment of craniosynostosis--is it the future? J Craniofac Surg 2012; 23(1): 225-8. [http://dx.doi.org/10.1097/SCS.0b013e318241b8f6] [PMID: 22337414]

[33]   Masserano B, Woo AS, Skolnick GB, *et al.* The temporal region in unilateral coronal craniosynostosis: fronto-orbital advancement versus endoscopy-assisted strip craniectomy. Cleft Palate Craniofac J 2018; 55(3): 423-9. [http://dx.doi.org/10.1177/1055665617739000] [PMID: 29437517]

[34]   Le MB, Patel K, Skolnick G, *et al.* Assessing long-term outcomes of open and endoscopic sagittal synostosis reconstruction using three-dimensional photography. J Craniofac Surg 2014; 25(2): 573-6. [http://dx.doi.org/10.1097/SCS.0000000000000613] [PMID: 24577302]

[35]   Zubovic E, Lapidus JB, Skolnick GB, Naidoo SD, Smyth MD, Patel KB. Cost comparison of surgical management of nonsagittal synostosis: traditional open versus endoscope-assisted techniques. J Neurosurg Pediatr 2020; 25(4): 351-60. [http://dx.doi.org/10.3171/2019.11.PEDS19515] [PMID: 31923895]

[36]   Riordan CP, Zurakowski D, Meier PM, Alexopoulos G, Meara JG, Proctor MR, *et al.* Minimally invasive endoscopic surgery for infantile craniosynostosis: a longitudinal cohort study. The Journal of pediatrics 2020; 216: 142-9. [http://dx.doi.org/10.1016/j.jpeds.2019.09.037]

[37]   Sanger C, David L, Argenta L. Latest trends in minimally invasive synostosis surgery. Curr Opin Otolaryngol Head Neck Surg 2014; 22(4): 316-21. [http://dx.doi.org/10.1097/MOO.0000000000000069] [PMID: 24927379]

[38]   Chocron Y, Azzi AJ, Galli R, *et al.* Operative time as the predominant risk factor for transfusion requirements in nonsyndromic craniosynostosis repair. Plast Reconstr Surg Glob Open 2020; 8(1)e2592 [http://dx.doi.org/10.1097/GOX.0000000000002592] [PMID: 32095402]

[39]   Fernandez PG, Taicher BM, Goobie SM, *et al.* Predictors of transfusion outcomes in pediatric complex cranial vault reconstruction: a multicentre observational study from the Pediatric Craniofacial Collaborative Group. Can J Anaesth 2019; 66(5): 512-26. [http://dx.doi.org/10.1007/s12630-019-01307-w] [PMID: 30767183]

[40]   Ali A, Basaran B, Yornuk M, *et al.* Factors influencing blood loss and postoperative morbidity in children undergoing craniosynostosis surgery: a retrospective study. Pediatr Neurosurg 2013; 49(6): 339-46. [http://dx.doi.org/10.1159/000368781] [PMID: 25472759]

[41]   Wolfswinkel EM, Howell LK, Fahradyan A, Azadgoli B, McComb JG, Urata MM. Is postoperative intensive care unit care necessary following cranial vault remodeling for sagittal synostosis? Plast Reconstr Surg 2017; 140(6): 1235-9. [http://dx.doi.org/10.1097/PRS.0000000000003848] [PMID: 29176416]

[42]   Chocron Y, Azzi A, Galli R, *et al.* Routine Postoperative Admission to the Intensive Care Unit Following Repair of Nonsyndromic Craniosynostosis: Is it Necessary? J Craniofac Surg 2019; 30(6): 1631-4. [http://dx.doi.org/10.1097/SCS.0000000000005327] [PMID: 30921065]

[43]   Gerety PA, Basta MN, Fischer JP, Taylor JA. Operative management of nonsyndromic sagittal synostosis: a headto-head meta-analysis of outcomes comparing 3 techniques. J Craniofac Surg 2015; 26(4): 1251-7.
[http://dx.doi.org/10.1097/SCS.0000000000001651] [PMID: 26080168]

[44]   Yan H, Abel TJ, Alotaibi NM, *et al.* A systematic review of endoscopic versus open treatment of craniosynostosis. Part 2: the nonsagittal single sutures. J Neurosurg Pediatr 2018; 22(4): 361-8.
[http://dx.doi.org/10.3171/2018.4.PEDS17730] [PMID: 29979132]

[45]   Farber SJ, Nguyen DC, Skolnick GB, Naidoo SD, Smyth MD, Patel KB. Anthropometric outcome measures in patients with metopic craniosynostosis. J Craniofac Surg 2017; 28(3): 713-6.
[http://dx.doi.org/10.1097/SCS.0000000000003495] [PMID: 28468154]

[46]   Nguyen DC, Patel KB, Skolnick GB, *et al.* Are endoscopic and open treatments of metopic synostosis equivalent in treating trigonocephaly and hypotelorism? J Craniofac Surg 2015; 26(1): 129-34.
[http://dx.doi.org/10.1097/SCS.0000000000001321] [PMID: 25534056]

[47]   Zubovic E, Woo AS, Skolnick GB, Naidoo SD, Smyth MD, Patel KB. Cranial base and posterior cranial vault asymmetry after open and endoscopic repair of isolated lambdoid craniosynostosis. J Craniofac Surg 2015; 26(5): 1568-73.
[http://dx.doi.org/10.1097/SCS.0000000000001891] [PMID: 26114505]

[48]   Runyan CM, Gabrick KS, Park JG, *et al.* Long-term outcomes of spring-assisted surgery for sagittal craniosynostosis. Plast Reconstr Surg 2020; 146(4): 833-41.
[http://dx.doi.org/10.1097/PRS.0000000000007168] [PMID: 32590513]

[49]   van Veelen MLC, Mathijssen IMJ. Spring-assisted correction of sagittal suture synostosis. Childs Nerv Syst 2012; 28(9): 1347-51.
[http://dx.doi.org/10.1007/s00381-012-1850-5] [PMID: 22872247]

[50]   Thwin M, Schultz TJ, Anderson PJ. Morphological, functional and neurological outcomes of craniectomy versus cranial vault remodeling for isolated nonsyndromic synostosis of the sagittal suture: a systematic review. JBI Database Syst Rev Implement Reports 2015; 13(9): 309-68.
[http://dx.doi.org/10.11124/01938924-201513090-00021] [PMID: 26470674]

[51]   Al-Shaqsi SZ, Rai A, Forrest C, Phillips J. Public perception of a normal head shape in children with sagittal craniosynostosis. J Craniofac Surg 2020; 31(4): 940-4.
[http://dx.doi.org/10.1097/SCS.0000000000006260] [PMID: 32149974]

[52]   Vogel TW, Woo AS, Kane AA, Patel KB, Naidoo SD, Smyth MD. A comparison of costs associated with endoscope-assisted craniectomy versus open cranial vault repair for infants with sagittal synostosis. J Neurosurg Pediatr 2014; 13(3): 324-31.
[http://dx.doi.org/10.3171/2013.12.PEDS13320] [PMID: 24410127]

[53]   Whitaker LA, Bartlett SP, Schut L, Bruce D. Craniosynostosis. Plast Reconstr Surg 1987; 80(2): 195-206.
[http://dx.doi.org/10.1097/00006534-198708000-00006] [PMID: 3602170]

[54]   Braun TL, Eisemann BS, Olorunnipa O, Buchanan EP, Monson LA. Safety outcomes in endoscopic versus open repair of metopic craniosynostosis. J Craniofac Surg 2018; 29(4): 856-60.
[http://dx.doi.org/10.1097/SCS.0000000000004299] [PMID: 29461368]

[55]   Ajami S, Rodriguez-Florez N, Ong J, *et al.* Mechanical and morphological properties of parietal bone in patients with sagittal craniosynostosis. J Mech Behav Biomed Mater 2022; 125104929
[http://dx.doi.org/10.1016/j.jmbbm.2021.104929] [PMID: 34773914]

[56]   Li Z, Park BK, Liu W, *et al.* A statistical skull geometry model for children 0-3 years old. PLoS One 2015; 10(5)e0127322
[http://dx.doi.org/10.1371/journal.pone.0127322] [PMID: 25992998]

CHAPTER 9

Autonomic Dysreflexia with Hypertension Following Durotomy-Related Intradural Spread of Irrigation Fluid and Air During Spinal Endoscopy

Roth A.A. Vargas[1,*], **Morgan P. Lorio**[2], **Paulo Sérgio Teixeira de Carvalho**[3], **Anthony Yeung**[4] and **Kai-Uwe Lewandrowski**[5,6,7]

[1] *Department of Neurosurgery, Foundation Hospital Centro Médico Campinas, Campinas SP, Brazil*

[2] *Advanced Orthopedics, 499 East Central Parkway, Altamonte Springs, FL 32701, USA*

[3] *Pain and Spine Minimally Invasive Surgery Service at Gaffre e Guinle University Hospital, Rio de Janeiro, Brazil*

[4] *Desert Institute for Spine Care, Phoenix, AZ, USA*

[5] *Center for Advanced Spine Care of Southern Arizona and Surgical Institute of Tucson, Tucson, AZ, USA*

[6] *Departmemt of Orthopaedics, Fundación Universitaria Sanitas, Bogotá, D.C., Colombia*

[7] *Department of Neurosurgery in the Video-Endoscopic Postgraduate Program at the Universidade Federal do Estado do Rio de Janeiro - UNIRIO, Rio de Janeiro, Brazil*

Abstract: Trivialization of durotomy can cause complications for endoscopic spine surgeons when a patient's neurological or cardiovascular status unexpectedly deteriorates during or after surgery. The literature on fluid management strategies, irrigation-related risk factors, and clinical consequences of incidental durotomy during spinal endoscopy is limited. However, it suggests that most patients can be managed with supportive care without formal dural repair. There is currently no validated irrigation protocol for endoscopic spine surgery. In this chapter, the authors report severe complications in several patients, including the spread of irrigation fluid, blood, and air into the intradural and intracranial spaces. They concluded that patients should be informed about the risks associated with irrigated spinal endoscopy before surgery. Infrequent yet not insignificant, adversities encompassing intracranial hemorrhage, hydrocephalus, cephalalgia, cervical discomfort, convulsive events, and the perilous autonomic dysreflexia manifesting as hypertensive episodes can transpire should the irrigation fluid inadvertently enter the spinal cord or dural sac. Adept endoscopic spinal surgeons postulate an association between durotomy events and equilibration pressures associated with irrigation, a conjunction that, when amalgamated with copious irrigation volumes, may prove disconcerting. Further research is needed to determine whether specific thresholds for pressure, flow, and total volume of irrigation fluid

---

[*] **Corresponding author Roth A.A. Vargas:** Department of Neurosurgery, Foundation Hospital Centro Médico Campinas, Campinas SP, Brazil; E-mail: rothvargas@hotmail.com

should be established and to identify any additional risk factors beyond incidental durotomy or prolonged surgery time.

Keywords: Lumbar endoscopic surgery, Irrigation flow- and pressure, Adverse events and complications.

INTRODUCTION

The use of irrigation during spinal endoscopy in patients with incidental durotomy has been associated with anecdotal evidence of adverse events and complications. This minimally invasive surgical approach has gained popularity among a new generation of spine surgeons, who now incorporate endoscopic procedures into their training programs [1 - 4]. Key opinion leaders in the field stress the importance of mastering the learning curve to achieve good clinical outcomes [5]. Training and credentialing standards are still evolving, and there is an ongoing debate about who should perform these minimally invasive spine operations [1, 3, 6]. As the number of endoscopic spine surgeries increases, so does the awareness of potential pitfalls, pearls, and complications specific to these procedures [7 - 9].

The investigators in this study suspected that the rate of unrecognized durotomy could be higher than the previously reported 1% [9]. They observed rare but severe neurological and cardiovascular complications in endoscopic spine surgery patients and attributed them to durotomy [10, 11]. To investigate further, they conducted epidural pressure measurements and surveyed endoscopic spine surgeons regarding irrigation-related adverse events and complications [10].

During surgery, the clear irrigation fluid makes it difficult for the surgeon to assess its flow pattern and direction. Limited and indirect observations can be made, such as monitoring the quantity and direction of bleeding from epidural vessels or the movement of intrathecal rootlets within the semi-transparent nerve sac. Observing the flow patterns of blood leaking from small epidural vessels provides valuable information about the flow direction, similar to studying dye injectors in aero- or fluid-dynamics studies. Other signs can also be helpful, such as the direction and extent of rootlet herniations through an incidental durotomy or annular fibers through an annular tear.

The literature on fluid management and irrigation-related problems during lumbar spinal endoscopy is limited. Consequently, the authors report on profound complications within a concise cohort of patients, ascribed to the inadvertent intradural dispersion of irrigation fluid consequent to unanticipated durotomy. Additionally, they convey findings from intraoperative measurements of epidural pressures garnered at the locus of surgical decompression. Moreover, the authors share the findings of a survey conducted among busy endoscopic spine surgeons, focusing on their usage patterns and perceived problems related to irrigation fluid. The authors aim to raise awareness among unsuspecting and novice endoscopic spine surgeons about the potential for sudden and unexpected declines in neurological and cardiovascular function, regardless of whether a durotomy is encountered when there is intradural spread of irrigation fluid.

Exemplary Problem Cases

The researchers observed durotomy-related complications during an irrigated spinal endoscopy in a 52-year-old female patient who underwent routine interlaminar C6/7 endoscopic decompression for persistent arm pain caused by disc herniation. Preoperative MRI scans indicated C6/7 posterolateral disc herniation with evident root compression. The surgery followed the technique described by Ruetten *et al.* (7-9), with the patient under general anesthesia and positioned prone. During the operation, controlling bleeding proved challenging, and a small 3-mm dural lesion was noted, possibly due to poor visualization caused by uncontrolled bleeding. The bleeding was successfully managed using bipolar coagulation, and dural repair was not deemed necessary following decompression (Figs. **1** and **2**).

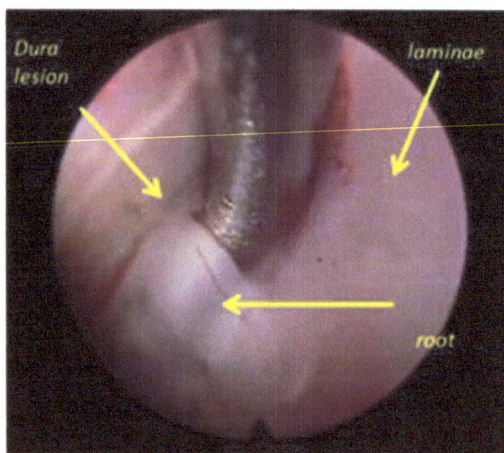

Fig. (1). In the illustrative case of a 52-year-old female who underwent a C6/7 disc herniation decompression *via* the interlaminar approach, fluid inadvertently permeated the intradural compartment through a minor unintentional durotomy. The hydrostatic pressure was augmented to enhance visual clarity. Following the procedure, the patient presented with diplopia and cephalalgia. Cranial computed tomography identified subarachnoid hemorrhage and hydrocephalus, consistent with Fischer Grade 4 subarachnoid bleeding.

After the surgery, the patient experienced postoperative symptoms, including neck pain, headache, and diplopia. Neurological examination revealed paresis of the right-sided lateral rectus muscle, suggesting abducens nerve paresis. Initially, motor weakness persisted in the right arm. A postoperative head CT scan revealed significant subarachnoid hemorrhage, hydrocephalus, and blood accumulation in various intracranial spaces, indicative of arterial Fisher Grade IV subarachnoid hemorrhage [12, 13]. Cerebral angiography conducted through femoral catheterization did not identify any aneurysms, angiomas, or other sources of intracranial bleeding. The patient received supportive care during a ten-day hospital stay, and her symptoms eventually resolved. Two male patients with incidental lumbar durotomy experienced intraoperative seizures, cardiac arrhythmia, and hypotension. One of these patients exhibited intracranial air entrapment on a head CT scan. Both patients were stabilized medically and discharged three days after the surgery.

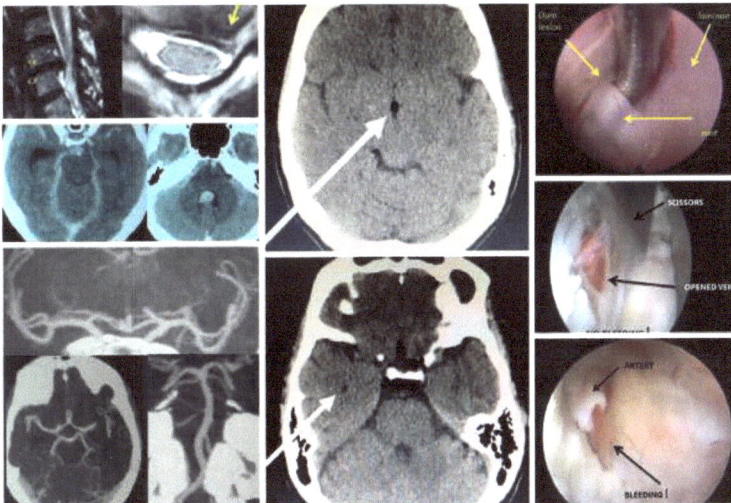

Fig. (2). Postoperative scans and videoendoscopic views of patients who experienced incidental durotomy and neurological complications following gravity irrigated-interlaminar full endoscopic spinal endoscopy. In the left column, postoperative sagittal and axial MRI scans of a 52-year-old female patient's cervical spine reveal hemorrhage spreading anteriorly and laterally, away from the posterior decompression site. A head CT scan showed significant blood accumulation in the subarachnoid space, basal cisterns III, IV, and lateral ventricles, and ventricular dilatation, indicating hydrocephalus. This condition was consistent with arterial subarachnoid Fisher grade IV hemorrhage. Notably, CT angiography *via* femoral catheterization did not identify any bleeding from potential vascular malformations like an aneurysm or angioma, suggesting that the blood traveled rostrally and intracranially with the irrigation fluid. In the center column, head CT scans of another male patient who underwent lumbar L4/5 interlaminar gravity-irrigated full endoscopic decompression surgery with an incidental lumbar durotomy are displayed. This patient experienced intraoperative seizures, cardiac arrhythmia, and hypotension. The head CT scan revealed the presence of intracranial air entrapment. Both patients shown were stabilized through appropriate medical intervention and were discharged from the hospital after ten and three days postoperatively, respectively. Images in the right column demonstrate an exemplary incidental lumbar durotomy identified in the second patient. In line with the observed pressure gradients, injury to an epidural vein typically results in less bleeding than an injured arterial vessel. Source: Reproduced under open access Creative Commons Attribution (CC BY) license (https://creativecommons.org/licenses/by/4.0/) from Vargas *et al.*, 2023 [10].

Endoscopic Technique

During the management of lumbar disc herniation and concomitant lateral recess stenosis, the interlaminar approach was adopted [14 - 16]. The patient was oriented in the prone orientation and prepped in accordance with established surgical standards. Anatomical landmarks within the cervical and lumbar spine, such as the midline, interlaminar window, intervertebral disc space, and facet joints, were demarcated utilizing intraoperative anteroposterior (PA) and lateral radiographs. After ascertaining the precise entry trajectories and inclinations, informed by the anatomical locale, dimension, and interrelations, a succinct incision was executed, typically distanced 2 to 3 cm from the median, targeting the facet joint. The RIWO VERTEBRIS™ lumbar apparatus equipped with a 30-degree optic was harnessed by the authors to access the posterior interlaminar aperture. Direct guidance of dilators to the ligamentum flavum was achieved with minimal reliance on fluoroscopic guidance, circumventing needle usage. Subsequent to positioning the working sheath atop the dilator, the intervention was executed employing a high-definition spinal endoscope furnished with a 30-degree perspective paired with uninterrupted gravity-facilitated irrigation.

The system's architecture was meticulously crafted to furnish paramount instrument efficacy, coupled with superior visual acuity, empowering the authors to swiftly detect even small durotomies. The endoscopic tools and powered burrs, integral to the procedure, boasted a slender design, mitigating undue trauma to the soft tissue matrix, ligamentum flavum, and neural entities. The operative strategy encompassed the amplification of the interlaminar aperture *via* a powered burr and the undertaking of a laminotomy at the posterior juncture of the rostral lamina. Typically, a partial excision of the inferior articular process (IAP) becomes imperative to garner access to the ligamentum flavum. Blunt dissection is employed to breach the ligamentum flavum, which is subsequently excised employing endoscopic pincers and a Kerrison rongeur. Neural components are delicately displaced, and any disc protrusion or other bony or pliable tissue stenosis is assiduously excised. Hemostasis and the attenuation of frayed soft tissues are achievable with a radiofrequency instrument. Post decompression, the cannula's orientation is modulated to offer a clear view of neural elements, and tactile affirmation of the decompression is secured through the employment of a neural probe.

Epidural Pressures

Under typical conditions, epidural pressures at baseline and intraoperatively exhibit variability contingent upon the prevailing clinical context and patient-specific attributes. In a quiescent state, accepted epidural pressures oscillate between 5 and 20 mm Hg [17]. In the milieu of spinal surgical intervention, these pressures may escalate, influenced by dynamics such as surgical tissue manipulation, introduction of irrigation fluid, and alterations in patient orientation. Existing literature cites a broad spectrum of intraoperative epidural pressures spanning 10 to 40 mm Hg. It behooves the surgical practitioner to assiduously monitor these pressures in real-time, ensuring confinement within permissible limits and promptly intervening upon discerning substantial elevations that potentiate complications. Notwithstanding, the pressing need persists for comprehensive research endeavors to delineate precise parameters and directives for judicious management of epidural pressures during spinal endoscopy.

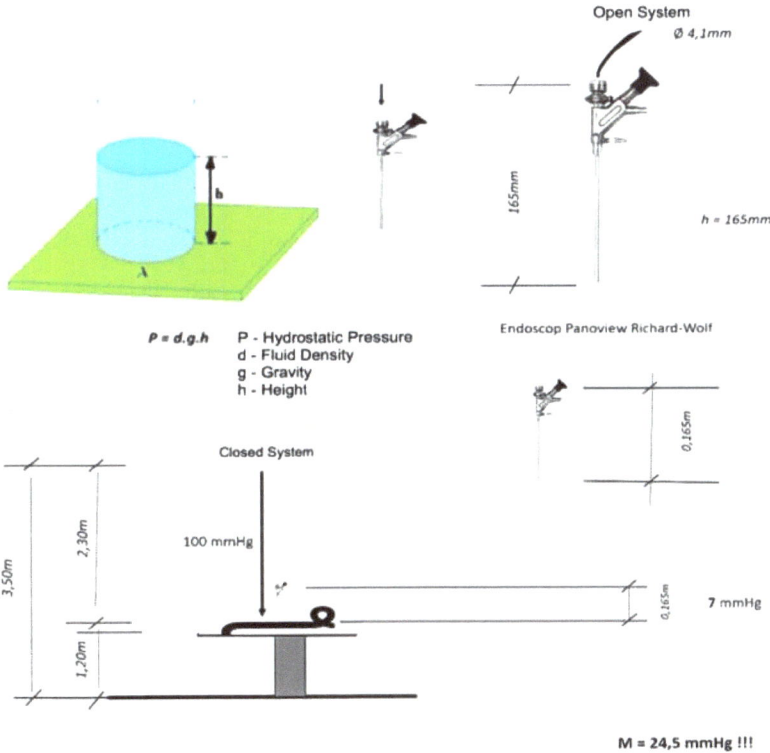

Fig. (3). The hydrostatic pressure within a static fluid column is principally dictated by the altitude of the liquid column, the intrinsic viscosity or density of the fluid, and gravitational forces. Notably, this pressure remains unaffected by the column's geometric attributes. In the course of full endoscopic lumbar spinal interventions, the research team executed precise intraoperative hydrostatic pressure determinations. Physiological saline reservoirs, each holding two liters, were strategically elevated to 2.30 meters above the patient, factoring in the stature of the operative platform. This configuration ensured the reservoirs' placement at an altitude of 3.50 meters from the ground level. A flexible conduit adjoined these reservoirs to the endoscope (Panoview Plus™ 25°, span 165mm, operational conduit Ø 4.1mm Richard-Wolf Vertebris™) *via* a bi-directional interface. The Baxter transducer apparatus was aligned at an equivalent elevation to the saline reservoirs, 3.50 meters superior to the ground. To sustain an unwavering hydrostatic pressure column during evaluations, the incorporation of an irrigation pump was deliberately omitted. Source: Reproduced under

Hydrostatic Epidural Measurements

Epidural pressure determinations were executed utilizing a Baxter bi-directional arterial line kit in conjunction with a transducer assembly introduced *via* the endoscopic conduit of the RIWO Spine Panoview Plus™ and Vertebris™ endoscope, targeting the spinal decompression locus. These pressure evaluations encompassed 12 patients who underwent standard endoscopic discectomy procedures at the intervertebral sites L4/5 and L5/S1. Employing a gravity-driven mechanism—sans an irrigation pump—the fluid reservoirs were strategically situated 2.3 meters superior to the patient's plane (Refer to Fig. **3**). In extrapolating the data, the authors postulated the potential implications of the Venturi phenomenon, elucidating the anticipated decrement in fluid pressure as it traverses a narrowed conduit segment (or choke) (See Fig. **2**). Within our gravity-propelled fluid irrigation framework, a decline in downstream pressure would theoretically augment fluid velocity, contingent upon fluid compression dynamics.

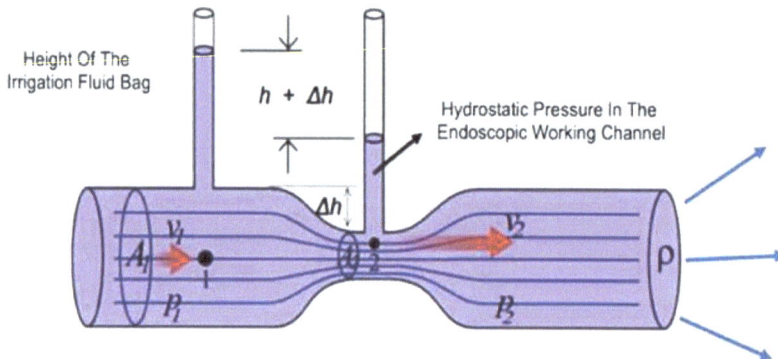

Fig. (4). The observed hydrostatic pressure differential, demarcated between the posterior aspect of the patient (103mmHg) and the median epidural pressure recorded at 24.5mmHg, is illustrative. This variance can be ascribed to the manifestation of the Venturi phenomenon. This dynamic is typified by a decrement in fluidic pressure as it traverses a narrowed or bottlenecked segment of a conduit. Within the canonical gravitational-assisted conduit configuration for spinal endoscopy, such a phenomenon is instigated as the fluid journeys from the primary tubing assembly into the slender irrigation passage of the spinal endoscope and subsequently into the epidural compartment. Following this, the fluid effluxes *via* the more expansive operational channel of the endoscope (Ø 4.1mm). This architectural layout necessitates multifarious alterations in diameter as the fluid navigates the system and the fluidic velocity verges on sonic speeds. Under circumstances where the fluidic architecture is experiencing a choked flow state, any further diminution in the succeeding pressure milieu will not augment velocity, barring situations where the fluid undergoes compression.

During intraoperative epidural hydrostatic pressure measurements at the endoscopic decompression locus, a lucid catheter, measuring 1.8 mm in diameter and equipped with three lateral apertures, was meticulously inserted through the endoscopic conduit. This catheter was deliberately situated in proximity to the surgical apparatus designated for herniated disc remediation. To streamline the evaluative process, an epidural/arterial catheter was linked to an Abbott Medex Disposable IBP Transducer (#IP-MX-300), subsequently interfaced with a Dräger Perseus A500 anesthetic machinery, complete with a visual display. Post-decompression, the catheter's position was adjusted adjacent to the dural sac or, if identified, in immediate juxtaposition to any dural perforation (Illustrated in Fig. **4**). Repetitive pressure assessments were undertaken, a minimum of thrice, within the identical decompression region, aiming to discern potential thermal shifts instigated by the radiofrequency instrument on the epidural hydrostatic pressures. Such evaluations transpired both in the presence and absence of the radiofrequency instrument's engagement. Documented pressure metrics were subsequently transcribed and manually integrated into a digital Excel database.

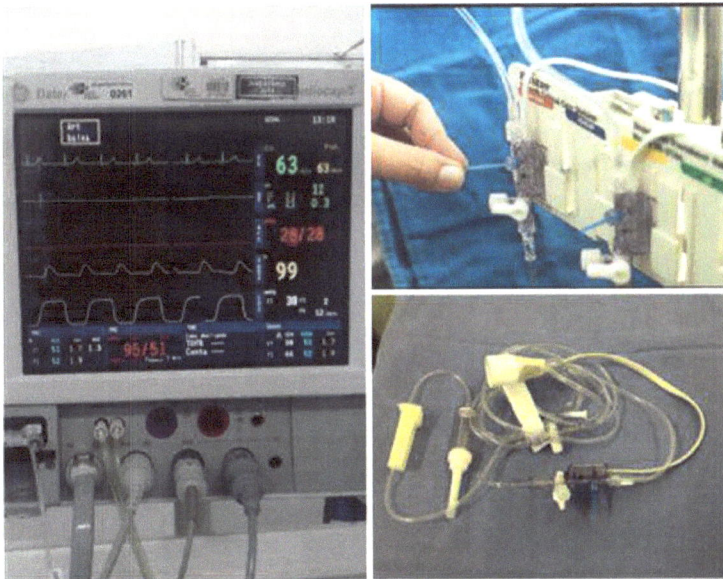

Fig. (5). A prototypical hydrostatic epidural pressure measurement configuration is depicted. Within this schema, a lucid catheter, boasting a 1.8 mm diameter and a trio of lateral apertures, was integrated *via* the endoscopic conduit at the locus of decompression. This catheter was meticulously aligned proximate to the surgical implement designated for the herniated disc amelioration. In a bid to streamline the quantification process, the epidural/arterial catheter was interfaced with an Abbott Medex Disposable IBP Transducer (#IP-MX-300). This was sequentially interfaced with a Dräger Perseus A500 anesthetic apparatus, complemented by a monitor.

Hydrostatic epidural pressure metrics are delineated in Table **1**. These pressure values were derived from 12 patients undergoing standard procedures at the L4/5 and L5/S1 interstices (Fig. **5**). The recorded pressures within the epidural domain oscillated between 20.0 and 29 mm Hg, with a median convergence at 24.5 mm Hg. By juxtaposition, the hydrostatic impetus conveyed to the endoscope *via* the gravimetrically-driven irrigation mechanism, from an aggregate elevation of 3.5 meters to the patient's altitude of 1.2 meters, had a mean of 103 mm Hg. Such data highlight a pronounced attenuation of 78.5 mm Hg from the inaugural hydrostatic measure at the patient's echelon prior to its transition into the spinal endoscope, culminating at 24.5 mm Hg in the epidural enclave.

Table 1. **Hydrostatic epidural pressure measurements in patients who underwent routine L4/5 and L5/S1 interlaminar full endoscopic discectomy.**

	Gender	Age	Weight	Measured Hydrostatic Pressure
1	M	54	82	26.5
2	M	62	71	20.0
3	F	46	131	22.5
4	M	65	92	26.0
5	M	72	86	23.0
6	F	58	61	29.0
7	F	51	65	20.0
8	F	46	90	28.0
9	M	39	78	23.5
10	M	40	89	21.0
11	M	36	70	29.0
12	M	52	62	25.5

DISCUSSION

Endoscopic spinal interventions, although increasingly favored beyond lumbar considerations, present unique challenges in the thoracic spine, particularly concerning the intricate vascular network servicing the spinal cord, primarily orchestrated *via* a triad of principal arteries. The anterior spinal artery is entrusted with perfusing the anterior spinal cord's two-thirds, whilst a duet of posterolateral spinal arteries caters to the posterior third's demands [18, 19]. The chief vascular conduit, denoted as the anterior spinal artery, emerges conjointly from the bilateral vertebral arteries proximate to the foramen magnum, augmented by segmental medullary vessels hailing from the aorta at each vertebral juncture [19]. Of these, the artery of Adamkiewicz stands prominent, alternatively recognized as arteria radicularis magna or the eminent anterior radiculomedullary artery [20]. The artery of Adamkiewicz's trajectory can be retraced to its provenance from the descending thoracic aorta, wherein a cadre of 8 to 10 intercostal and lumbar arterioles bifurcate antero-posteriorly [21]. The posterior offshoots yield the radiculomedullary artery, musculature-related vessels, and dorsal somatic branches. The cardinal radiculomedullary artery further dichotomizes into a dominant anterior and a diminutive posterior counterpart, with the artery of Adamkiewicz reigning as the preeminent anterior radiculomedullary artery. As this artery penetrates the intervertebral foramen, its location typically mirrors, occasionally anterior to, the egressing thoracic nerve, adopting a slightly craniolateral course in tandem with the ventral root and the anterior spinal cord facade [19]. On its ascendant course, the artery of Adamkiewicz etches a distinctive "hairpin" configuration on angiographic portrayals as it affiliates with the anterior spinal artery [22 - 24].

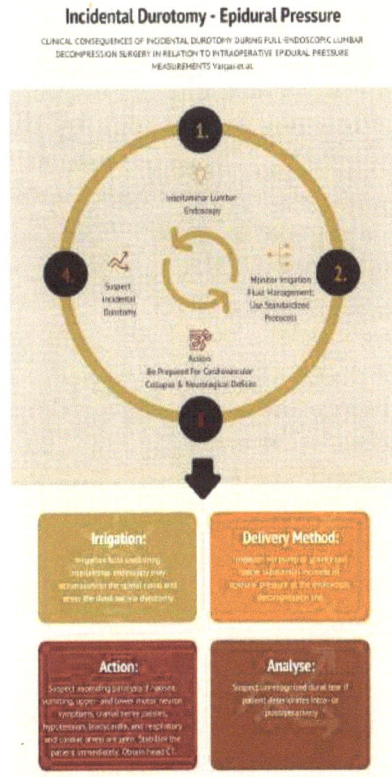

Fig. (6). Infogramm on the protocol on how to deal with unexpected postoperative clinical course suspicious of irrigation-related problems in patients with suspected incidental durotomy.

Utilizing coagulation during transforaminal neuroforaminal access, often harnessed to mitigate hemorrhage and enhance visualization, poses noteworthy perils. Given the grave implications, the authors predominantly advocate for a laterally-skewed interlaminar trajectory, furnishing a direct conduit to the facet joint recess. Nonetheless, the transforaminal modality might present a more apt choice for patients manifesting pronounced myelopathy due to a centrally-situated, ossified herniation underscored by myelomalacia on thoracic MRI evaluations. Such ossified central protrusions emerge as the foremost challenge in thoracic endoscopy. The transforaminal strategy curtails the probability of undue spinal cord handling or retraction, emphasizing the intervertebral disc beneath the dural sac. This can proffer a viable counterpart to the interlaminar technique, especially once the locus of the AKA system has been demarcated *via* CTA, thereby obviating indiscriminate coagulation of the foraminal root vasculature.

CONCLUSION

We emphatically endorse the inclusion of a rigorous computed tomography angiography (CTA) assessment to delineate the Adamkiewicz arterial network and verify its ingress point into the thoracic vertebral canal before thoracic endoscopic discectomy. An adverse incident, wherein a patient succumbed to postoperative paraplegia, catalyzed this modification in the preoperative diagnostic regimen, resonating deeply with the patient, their kin, and the medical cadre. The CTA imaging protocols employed for this inquiry, as previously described, have garnered widespread adoption [25, 26]. The comparative efficacy of magnetic resonance angiography (MRA) juxtaposed with CTA for scrutinizing the Adamkiewicz architecture is presently under rigorous investigation [24]. Acknowledging that the Adamkiewicz artery might be non-existent in roughly 10% of the population, it becomes imperative for the interpreting radiologist to assiduously delineate the intercostal vessels during the arterial examination, often synchronized with the radicular arteries' contrast enhancement [25, 27]. Any deviation from this stringent radiological protocol might obfuscate the unequivocal identification of the Adamkiewicz artery's presence or lack thereof. The authors highlight the paramountcy of this methodological fidelity in endoscopic spinal operations across the thoracolumbar junction.

REFERENCES

[1]   Lewandrowski KU, Bergamashi JP, Telfeian AE, de Carvalho PST, Leon JFR. Training and Credentialing Standards for Minimally Invasive Spinal Surgery Techniques: Results of a SurveyBACKGROUND: The controversy continues on how to best become proficient in contemporary minimally invasive spinal surgery techniques (MISST). Postgrad Pain Physician 2023; 26(1): 29-37.

[2] Lewandrowski KU, Elfar JC, Li ZM, *et al.* The Changing Environment in Postgraduate Education in Orthopedic Surgery and Neurosurgery and Its Impact on Technology-Driven Targeted Interventional and Surgical Pain Management: Perspectives from Europe, Latin America, Asia, and The United States. J Pers Med 2023; 13(5): 852.
[http://dx.doi.org/10.3390/jpm13050852] [PMID: 37241022]

[3] Lewandrowski KU, Soriano-Sánchez JA, Zhang X, *et al.* Surgeon training and clinical implementation of spinal endoscopy in routine practice: results of a global survey. J Spine Surg 2020; 6(S1) (Suppl. 1): S237-48.
[http://dx.doi.org/10.21037/jss.2019.09.32] [PMID: 32195431]

[4] Lewandrowski KU, Soriano-Sánchez JA, Zhang X, *et al.* Surgeon motivation, and obstacles to the implementation of minimally invasive spinal surgery techniques. J Spine Surg 2020; 6(S1) (Suppl. 1): S249-59.
[http://dx.doi.org/10.21037/jss.2019.08.02] [PMID: 32195432]

[5] Lewandrowski KU, Telfeian AE, Hellinger S, *et al.* Difficulties, Challenges, and the Learning Curve of Avoiding Complications in Lumbar Endoscopic Spine Surgery. Int J Spine Surg 2021; 15 (Suppl. 3): S21-37.
[http://dx.doi.org/10.14444/8161] [PMID: 34974418]

[6] Yeung AT, Roberts A, Shin P, Rivers E, Paterson A, Paterson A. Suggestions for a Practical and Progressive Approach to Endoscopic Spine Surgery Training and Privileges. J Spine 2018; 7(2)
[http://dx.doi.org/10.4172/2165-7939.1000414]

[7] Lewandrowski KU. Incidence, Management, and Cost of Complications After Transforaminal Endoscopic Decompression Surgery for Lumbar Foraminal and Lateral Recess Stenosis: A Value Proposition for Outpatient Ambulatory Surgery. Int J Spine Surg 2019; 13(1): 53-67.
[http://dx.doi.org/10.14444/6008] [PMID: 30805287]

[8] Lewandrowski KU, Dowling Á, Calderaro AL, *et al.* Dysethesia due to irritation of the dorsal root ganglion following lumbar transforaminal endoscopy: Analysis of frequency and contributing factors. Clin Neurol Neurosurg 2020; 197: 106073.
[http://dx.doi.org/10.1016/j.clineuro.2020.106073] [PMID: 32683194]

[9] Lewandrowski KU, Hellinger S, De Carvalho PST, *et al.* Dural Tears During Lumbar Spinal Endoscopy: Surgeon Skill, Training, Incidence, Risk Factors, and Management. Int J Spine Surg 2021; 15(2): 280-94.
[http://dx.doi.org/10.14444/8038] [PMID: 33900986]

[10] Vargas RAA, Hagel V, Xifeng Z, *et al.* Durotomy- and Irrigation-Related Serious Adverse Events During Spinal Endoscopy: Illustrative Case Series and International Surgeon Survey. Int J Spine Surg 2023; 17(3): 387-98.
[http://dx.doi.org/10.14444/8454] [PMID: 37315993]

[11] Vargas RAA, Moscatelli M, Vaz de Lima M, *et al.* Clinical Consequences of Incidental Durotomy during Full-Endoscopic Lumbar Decompression Surgery in Relation to Intraoperative Epidural Pressure Measurements. J Pers Med 2023; 13(3): 381.
[http://dx.doi.org/10.3390/jpm13030381] [PMID: 36983563]

[12] Fisher CM, Kistler JP, Davis JM. Relation of cerebral vasospasm to subarachnoid hemorrhage visualized by computerized tomographic scanning. Neurosurgery 1980; 6(1): 1-9.
[http://dx.doi.org/10.1227/00006123-198001000-00001] [PMID: 7354892]

[13] Rosen DS, Macdonald RL. Subarachnoid hemorrhage grading scales: a systematic review. Neurocrit Care 2005; 2(2): 110-8.
[http://dx.doi.org/10.1385/NCC:2:2:110] [PMID: 16159052]

[14] Wasinpongwanich K, Pongpirul K, Lwin KMM, Kesornsak W, Kuansongtham V, Ruetten S. Full-Endoscopic Interlaminar Lumbar Discectomy: Retrospective Review of Clinical Results and Complications in 545 International Patients. World Neurosurg 2019; 132: c922-8.

[http://dx.doi.org/10.1016/j.wneu.2019.07.101] [PMID: 31326641]

[15]   Ruetten S, Komp M, Merk H, Godolias G. Full-endoscopic interlaminar and transforaminal lumbar discectomy *versus* conventional microsurgical technique: a prospective, randomized, controlled study. Spine 2008; 33(9): 931-9.
[http://dx.doi.org/10.1097/BRS.0b013e31816c8af7] [PMID: 18427312]

[16]   Ruetten S. Full-endoscopic Operations of the Spine in Disk Herniations and Spinal Stenosis. Surg Technol Int 2011; 21: 284-98.
[PMID: 22505003]

[17]   Hayek SM, Veizi E, Hanes M. Treatment-Limiting Complications of Percutaneous Spinal Cord Stimulator Implants: A Review of Eight Years of Experience From an Academic Center Database. Neuromodulation 2015; 18(7): 603-9.
[http://dx.doi.org/10.1111/ner.12312] [PMID: 26053499]

[18]   Klakeel M, Thompson J, Srinivasan R, Mcdonald F. Anterior spinal cord syndrome of unknown etiology. Proc Bayl Univ Med Cent 2015; 28(1): 85-7.
[http://dx.doi.org/10.1080/08998280.2015.11929201] [PMID: 25552812]

[19]   Bican O, Minagar A, Pruitt AA. The spinal cord: a review of functional neuroanatomy. Neurol Clin 2013; 31(1): 1-18.
[http://dx.doi.org/10.1016/j.ncl.2012.09.009] [PMID: 23186894]

[20]   Kroszczynski AC, Kohan K, Kurowski M, Olson TR, Downie SA. Intraforaminal location of thoracolumbar anterior medullary arteries. Pain Med 2013; 14(6): 808-12.
[http://dx.doi.org/10.1111/pme.12056] [PMID: 23438301]

[21]   Yadav N, Pendharkar H, Kulkarni GB. Spinal Cord Infarction: Clinical and Radiological Features. J Stroke Cerebrovasc Dis 2018; 27(10): 2810-21.
[http://dx.doi.org/10.1016/j.jstrokecerebrovasdis.2018.06.008] [PMID: 30093205]

[22]   Murthy NS, Maus TP, Behrns CL. Intraforaminal location of the great anterior radiculomedullary artery (artery of Adamkiewicz): a retrospective review. Pain Med 2010; 11(12): 1756-64.
[http://dx.doi.org/10.1111/j.1526-4637.2010.00948.x] [PMID: 21134118]

[23]   N'da HA, Chenin L, Capel C, Havet E, Le Gars D, Peltier J. Microsurgical anatomy of the Adamkiewicz artery–anterior spinal artery junction. Surg Radiol Anat 2016; 38(5): 563-7.
[http://dx.doi.org/10.1007/s00276-015-1596-3] [PMID: 26627692]

[24]   Yoshioka K, Niinuma H, Ehara S, Nakajima T, Nakamura M, Kawazoe K. MR angiography and CT angiography of the artery of Adamkiewicz: state of the art. Radiographics 2006; 26 (Suppl. 1): S63-73.
[http://dx.doi.org/10.1148/rg.26si065506] [PMID: 17050520]

[25]   Guziński M, Bryl M, Ziemińska K, Wolny K, Sąsiadek M, Garcarek J. Detection of the Adamkiewiczartery in computed tomography of the thorax and abdomen. Adv Clin Exp Med 2017; 26(1): 31-7.
[http://dx.doi.org/10.17219/acem/62788] [PMID: 28397429]

[26]   Theologis AA, Ramirez J, Diab M, Preoperative CT. Preoperative CT Angiography Informs Instrumentation in Anterior Spine Surgery for Idiopathic Scoliosis. J Am Acad Orthop Surg Glob Res Rev 2020; 4(4): e19.00123.
[http://dx.doi.org/10.5435/JAAOSGlobal-D-19-00123] [PMID: 32377614]

[27]   Lindeire S, Hauser JM. Anatomy, Back, Artery Of Adamkiewicz. Treasure Island (FL): StatPearls 2022.
[PMID: 30422566]

CHAPTER 10

Russian Roulette of Thoracic Spinal Endoscopy: The Importance of Preoperative Identification of Adamkiewicz System

Roth A.A. Vargas[1], Marco Moscatelli[2] and Kai-Uwe Lewandrowski[3,4,5,*]

[1] *Department of Neurosurgery, Foundation Hospital Centro Médico Campinas, Campinas SP, Brazil*

[2] *Clinica NeuroLife, Natal, RN, Brazil*

[3] *Center for Advanced Spine Care of Southern Arizona and Surgical Institute of Tucson, Tucson, AZ, USA*

[4] *Departmemt of Orthopaedics, Fundación Universitaria Sanitas, Bogotá, D.C., Colombia*

[5] *Department of Neurosurgery in the Video-Endoscopic Postgraduate Program at the Universidade Federal do Estado do Rio de Janeiro - UNIRIO, Rio de Janeiro, Brazil*

Abstract: Thoracic endoscopic spine surgery is gaining traction. During thoracic decompression, the arterial Adamkewicz system (AKA) can be encountered, with potentially severe implications if injured. This chapter outlines a diagnostic protocol and patient selection for the surgery based on a study examining surgical risks tied to the radicular magna artery. The authors share insights from fifteen patients with thoracic herniated discs and spinal stenosis who underwent preoperative CTA. This assessed the anatomical relationship of the Magna radicular artery to the surgical area. The Adamkiewicz artery's prevalent locations were T10/11 (15.4%), T11/12 (23.1%), and T9/10 (30.8%). Patients were grouped into three categories based on their pathology's proximity to the AKA foraminal entry. In five instances, the Magna radicular artery entered the spinal canal near the nerve root at the surgery site, prompting a surgical approach adjustment. The authors advocate for CTA evaluation to gauge surgical risks and adapt thoracic discectomy techniques based on the magna radicular artery's closeness to the pathology.

Keywords: Artery of Adamkiewicz, Spinal cord blood supply, Anterior spinal cord syndrome.

***Corresponding author Kai-Uwe Lewandrowski:** Center for Advanced Spine Care of Southern Arizona and Surgical Institute of Tucson, Tucson, AZ, USA; Departmemt of Orthopaedics, Fundación Universitaria Sanitas, Bogotá, D.C., Colombia and Department of Neurosurgery in the Video-Endoscopic Postgraduate Program at the Universidade Federal do Estado do Rio de Janeiro - UNIRIO, Rio de Janeiro, Brazil; E-mail: rothvargas@hotmail.com

Kai-Uwe Lewandrowski & William Omar Contreras López (Eds.)

INTRODUCTION

Thoracic endoscopic spine surgery is increasingly favored due to its minimally invasive characteristics and advantages over conventional methods such as laminectomy, costotransversectomy, and extracavitary interventions in the cervical and thoracic spine [1 - 3]. During thoracic procedures, whether open or endoscopic, segmental vessels, comprising arteries and veins, might be encountered, either traversing the disc space or appearing during decompression [4, 5]. When access to the herniated disc is challenging due to obstructions like the facet joint or rib head, vessel ligation might be an option [6]. This article's authors emphasize the importance of the arterial Adamkewicz system (AKA) in thoracic decompression and outline criteria for opting between contemporary, minimally invasive, encompassing endoscopic, and traditional surgical techniques [7].

The artery of Adamkiewicz, or Magna radicularis, displays variability in its positioning and trajectory within the thoracic spine [8]. While specialists are versed in the risks associated with standard thoracic interventions, the potential harm to the arterial network nourishing the thoracic spinal cord during endoscopy might be overlooked. Expertly executed spinal endoscopy can relieve pain from identified sources [9-15], but it's sometimes perceived as a basic operation not requiring specialized training [16, 17]. As a result, practitioners from diverse fields, like interventional radiology and pain management, undertake endoscopic decompressions with varied proficiency [18-24].

Underestimating the procedure, combined with its lower complications compared to open translaminar operations, might foster undue confidence [25]. However, compromising the Adamkiewicz system can yield grave outcomes, especially in settings like ambulatory centers without comprehensive support, leading to complications like paraplegia. In this manuscript, the authors detail their approach using the magna radicularis protocol for categorizing patients for thoracic disc procedures, either open or endoscopic. They discuss a retrospective analysis and their assessment framework for pinpointing the AKA's proximity to the surgical area before embarking on thoracic decompression.

Anatomical Variations

There are variations in the anatomical configuration of the AKA system. Typically, it originates from the left side of the aorta between the T8 and L2 levels, with the most common location being between T9 and T12. However, there have been reports of the AKA entering the spinal canal as low as the L2/3 level. The AKA was discovered incidentally after a patient experienced spinal cord infarction following a right-sided transforaminal epidural steroid injection

[25]. The authors recommended injecting at a lower position in the neuroforamen, just above the caudal pedicle, as a routine practice [25]. In approximately 15% of patients, the AKA is found at the T8 level, with a documented diameter ranging from 0.6 to 1.8 mm [7]. Other anatomical variations include the presence of more than one AKA or the AKA system arising from the right side of the aorta or outside the typical T8 through L2 range. Furthermore, the angle at which the AKA joins the anterior spinal artery system may vary [7]. In some cases, collateral circulation from the muscular, intercostal, or lumbar arteries may be present, especially if the AKA is occluded [25]. Injury to the AKA system can result in anterior spinal cord syndrome, characterized by motor deficits and typically preserved sensory function [26, 27]. Neurological damage may manifest as fecal and urinary incontinence.

AKA Identification

Computed tomography angiography (CTA) is recommended when assessing thoracoabdominal aortic aneurysm to pinpoint the AKA [28, 29]. In one instance, the authors identified its entry into the spinal canal at the planned thoracic surgical level in a patient (Fig. **1**) [28]. This finding led them to consistently employ CTA for those with thoracic disc herniation to avert potential neurological issues. When the surgical plan and the AKA's position align on the same side, there have been adjustments in surgical tactics, as documented in prior instances [30-33]. Differentiating the AKA from the anterior radiculomedullary vein is vital due to their parallel trajectories [34].

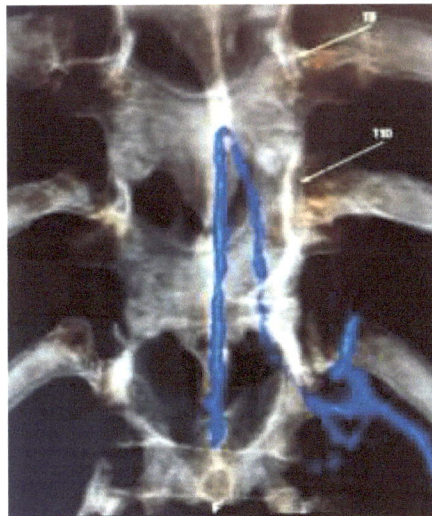

Fig. (1). Coronal computed Tomography (CT) angiography shows the entry foramen of the magna radicular artery and Adamkiewicz system.

Using the "continuity technique," the authors distinguished the radiculomedullary vein from the AKA by tracing the vessel to its origin in the aorta [35]. For gauging the risk of harming the AKA during surgery, they categorized the relationship between the AKA's entry point and the pressing symptomatic pathology into three classifications: Far type (significant distance between pathology and AKA), Near type (pathology close to, but not at, the AKA's entry point, possibly an adjacent level), and Foraminal type (pathology located in the AKA's entry foramen, deemed the riskiest).

Preoperative Planning

Before surgery, surgeons should determine whether the or transforaminal approach can effectively address the patient's compressive pathology. Situations with herniations that have moved significantly or bony issues distant from the thoracic disc space might be more apt for conventional open procedures, providing a wider view of the sensitive spinal cord. However, selecting the best surgical method should be a collaborative decision with the surgeon, taking into account their expertise and familiarity with endoscopic techniques. MRI, CT, and CTA scans are advisable, with the justification for CTA detailed subsequently.

Choice of Endoscopic Approach

The authors advocate for the posterior interlaminar method *via* the facet joint when performing endoscopic thoracic spine surgery. For clear visibility of the dural sac and the exiting nerve root, it's pivotal to carve out a broad interlaminar space with a drill. The decompression might entail either subtotal or full facetectomy, usually initiating with the inferior articular process (IAP). Even with significant decompression, the risk of iatrogenic instability is minimal, given the natural sturdiness of the thoracic spine and rib cage. Ruetten *et al.* recently suggested the transthoracic lateral retropleural method, underscoring the importance of coagulating or tying off the intercostal artery [6]. Nonetheless, these researchers didn't explicitly advise on preoperative pinpointing of the Magna radicular artery in this work or their other studies on full-endoscopic thoracic surgery [5, 6, 36].

Endoscopic Surgery Technique

The authors utilize a lateralized interlaminar approach for thoracic disc herniation, which offers direct access to the thoracic intervertebral disc and circumvents the rib head's attachment to the costovertebral joint. This method addresses potential obstructions posed by the rib head-disc relationship and ensures minimized collateral damage. Nonetheless, the accessible space is confined to the interlaminar window. This window permits yellow ligament resection and central spinal canal and lateral recess decompression. In instances with limited or no interlaminar window in the thoracic spine, significant lamina and lateral facet joint removal might be essential, employing a high-speed burr. The thoracolumbar spine's transforaminal endoscopy adheres to documented protocols [6, 24, 37-39].

For both methodologies, the patient is placed prone and prepped conventionally. Vital landmarks like the midline, interlaminar window, disc space, and facet joints are highlighted *via* intraoperative PA and lateral visuals. After determining attack angles and insertion sites, an incision is initiated – typically 3-5 cm off the midline for interlaminar and 6-7 cm laterally for transforaminal. Subsequent actions use lateral fluoroscopic monitoring and steady videoendoscopic visualization. Pinpointing the exact surgical level in thoracic operations, especially using intraoperative fluoroscopy, is complex, with an erroneous surgery rate of around 10%. Radiologist consultation is advisable during uncertainties. The working cannula, placed atop step-by-step dilators, is aligned where the facet joint connects with the lamina. A power drill crafts the interlaminar window, and the working cannula's beveled side faces the ligamentum flavum. Tools such as rongeurs, a radiofrequency probe, and burrs can expose the lamina's inferior lateral edge. As decompression proceeds, the working cannula shifts towards the lateral recess. Often, the facet joint on the approach side requires full extraction. After exposing the herniated disc, any dura and nerve root adhesions need detaching. After completing decompression, proper neural structure visualization is crucial, ensuring thorough decompression *via* palpation with a hook.

Inclusion and Exclusion Criteria

Eligibility for the thoracic discectomy procedure required patients to have persistent thoracic back or flank pain. To qualify, patients must have experienced symptoms for a minimum of six months despite three months of physiotherapy and adherence to recommended medical and interventional pain treatments. A comprehensive clinical assessment was conducted, highlighting signs of thoracic disc herniation, such as sensory loss, motor weakness, and upper motor neuron indicators. Diagnostic tools used encompassed standing X-rays, thoracic MRI, and CT scans, with a particular focus on CTA to assess the AKA system and its influence on tributaries at the operative thoracic spine level. The study excluded individuals with pre-existing neurological disorders or spinal cord compression elsewhere in the spine, affecting movement. Further disqualifications for endoscopic decompression were severe bony obstructions in the central canal or foramen, pronounced deformities over 40 degrees, conus medullaris syndrome, systemic neuropathy, spinal tumors, blood disorders, pregnancy, allergies, and cognitive or psychiatric conditions impacting communication or understanding.

Clinical Series

In the study, 15 patients with symptoms of thoracic disc herniation underwent endoscopic decompression after an incidental AKA finding in the first patient. Using a preoperative CTA protocol detailed later, the potential neurological risks from damaging the AKA system and resulting spinal cord ischemia were assessed. The cohort included 10 females (66.7%) and 5 males (33.3%), with ages averaging 58.53 ± 19.57 years, spanning from 31 to 89 years. On average, post-procedure monitoring lasted 30.13 ± 13.42 months.

The primary reason for surgery was continuous pain due to herniated nucleus pulposus (HNP) and foraminal stenosis. Table 1 provides data on the magna artery's entry point and laterality *via* CTA. Radiographic evidence confirmed the Adamkiewicz system in 93.33% (14 out of 15) of the patients, as detailed in Table 1. Notably, in a third of the study group (5 out of 15), the Magna radicularis was seen entering the spinal canal on the exiting nerve root's ventral surface *via* the neuroforamen at the operational level, prompting surgical approach adjustments.

Table 1. Foraminal entry level and side of the artery of Adamkiewicz.

Magna Level	Frequency	Percent	Cumulative Percent
L2/3	1	6.7	6.7
NOT IDENTIFIED	1	6.7	13.3
T10/11	3	20.0	33.3
T11/12	3	20.0	53.3
T12/L1	1	6.7	60.0
T7/8	1	6.7	66.7
T8/9	1	6.7	73.3
T9/10	4	26.7	100.0
Total	15	100.0	
SIDE	Frequency	Percent	Cumulative Percent
LEFT	7	46.7	46.7
NOT IDENTIFIED	1	6.7	6.7
RIGHT	7	46.7	46.7
Total	15	100.0	100.0

Table 2 details the surgical levels and corresponding painful pathologies for ease of comparison. Meanwhile, Table 3 offers insights into the surgical procedures and the challenges faced during them. Of the participants, eight had painful pathologies distant from the AKA's foraminal entry (type 1). Three were near this entry point (type 2), while four underwent decompression precisely at the foraminal entry (type 3). In 7 of these cases, the surgical point was either the same as or close to the AKA system's foraminal entry. Interestingly, in 5 of the 15 cases, the Magna radicularis was found to enter the spinal canal at the exiting nerve root's front side within the neuroforamen, leading to changes in surgical methodology.

Table 2. Surgical level and symptomatic pathology.

Surgical Level	Frequency	Percent	Cumulative Percent
T10/11 RIGHT	1	6.7	6.7
T11/12 RIGHT	1	6.7	13.3
T12/L1 CENTRAL	2	13.3	26.7
T4/5 LEFT	1	6.7	33.3
T5/6 LEFT	1	6.7	40.0
T5/6 RIGHT	1	6.7	46.7
T6/7 CENTRAL	1	6.7	53.3
T6/7 RIGHT	1	6.7	60.0
T7/8 LEFT	2	13.3	73.3
T7/8 RIGHT	1	6.7	80.0
T8/9 RIGHT	2	13.3	93.3
T9/10 LEFT	1	6.7	100.0
Total	15	100.0	
PATHOLOGY	Frequency	Percent	Cumulative Percent
BONY FORAMINAL STENOSIS	3	20.0	20.0
BURST FRACTURE WITH CORD COMPRESSION	1	6.7	26.7
CALCIFIED HNP	3	20.0	46.7
HNP	7	46.7	93.3
RETROLISTHESIS, DEFORMITY, NEUROFIBROMATOSIS	1	6.7	100.0
Total	15	100.0	

HNP – Herniated nucleus pulposus.

Table 3. Surgical treatment and encountered problems.

TREATMENT	Frequency	Percent	Cumulative Percent
COSTOTRANSVERSECTOMY	1	6.7	6.7
ENDOSCOPIC DECOMPRESSION	6	40.0	46.7
LAMINECTOMY & FORAMINOTOMY	1	6.7	53.3
LAMINECTOMY & FUSION	2	13.3	66.7
NON-SURGICAL / TESI	3	20.0	86.7
NON-SURGICAL TREATMENT	2	13.3	100.0
Total	15	100.0	
PROBLEM	Frequency	Percent	Cumulative Percent
N.A.	8	53.3	53.3
AV FISTULA	1	6.7	60.0
LARGE CALCIFIED CENTRAL HNP	2	13.3	73.3
MULTILEVEL SEVERE STENOSIS	1	6.7	80.0
NEUROFIBROMATOSIS, RETROLISTHESIS & DEFORMITY	1	6.7	86.7
POSTTRAUMATIC INSTABILITY	1	6.7	93.3
UNABLE TO FIND MAGNA	1	6.7	100.0
Total	15	100.0	

TESI – Transforaminal epidural steroid injection; HNP – Herniated nucleus pulposus.

Patients presenting with large centrally-located calcified herniated discs, pronounced or multilevel foraminal stenosis, burst fractures, deformities, or instability were not considered candidates for endoscopic decompression. These individuals underwent traditional open decompression procedures, either laminectomy or fusion, based on the specific pathology. If both open and endoscopic surgeries were deemed hazardous or unfeasible for some patients, they received interventional treatment using transforaminal epidural steroid injections (TESI) for their herniated disc-related pain.

Table **4** presents the clinical data of the study patients, including information about the magna and surgical level, encountered painful pathology, provided treatment, and encountered problems.

Table 4. Clinical data of thoracic discectomy patients with available AKA studies.

No	Magna Level	Magna Type	Magna Side	Surgical Level & Side	Pathology	Treatment	Problem
1	T9/10	1	RIGHT	T8/9 RIGHT	HNP	ENDOSCOPIC DECOMPRESSION	

(Table 4) cont.....

No	Magna Level	Magna Type	Magna Side	Surgical Level & Side	Pathology	Treatment	Problem
2	T8/9	1	LEFT	T5/6 RIGHT	BONY FORAMINAL STENOSIS	ENDOSCOPIC DECOMPRESSION	
3	T11/12	2	RIGHT	T6/7 CENTRAL	CALCIFIED HNP	NON-SURGICAL TREATMENT	AV FISTULA
4	L2/3	1	LEFT	T6/7 RIGHT	HNP	ENDOSCOPIC DECOMPRESSION	
5	T9/10	1	LEFT	T5/6 LEFT	HNP	NON-SURGICAL / TESI	
6	T10/11	1	RIGHT	T4/5 LEFT	HNP	NON-SURGICAL / TESI	
7	T11/12	3	LEFT	T12/L1 CENTRAL	RETROLISTHESIS, DEFORMITY	LAMINECTOMY & FUSION	NEUROFIBROMATOSIS, RETROLISTHESIS & DEFORMITY
8	T9/10	2	LEFT	T7/8 LEFT	CALCIFIED HNP	COSTOTRANS-VERSECTOMY	LARGE CALCIFIED CENTRAL HNP, PARAPLEGIA
9	T11/12	3	RIGHT	T11/12 RIGHT	CALCIFIED HNP	NON-SURGICAL / TESI	LARGE CALCIFIED CENTRAL HNP
10	NOT IDENTIFIED	1	NOT IDENTIFIED	T7/8 LEFT	HNP	ENDOSCOPIC DECOMPRESSION	UNABLE TO FIND MAGNA
11	T9/10	1	LEFT	T9/10 LEFT	BONY FORAMINAL STENOSIS	NON-SURGICAL TREATMENT	MULTILEVEL SEVERE STENOSIS
12	T12/L1	1	LEFT	T8/9 RIGHT	BONY FORAMINAL STENOSIS	LAMINECTOMY & FORAMINOTOMY	
13	T10/11	2	RIGHT	T12/L1 CENTRAL	BURST FRACTURE WITH CORD COMPRESSION	LAMINECTOMY & FUSION	POSTTRAUMATIC INSTABILITY
14	T10/11	3	RIGHT	T10/11 CENTRAL	HNP	ENDOSCOPIC DECOMPRESSION	
15	T7/8	3	RIGHT	T7/8 RIGHT	HNP	ENDOSCOPIC DECOMPRESSION	

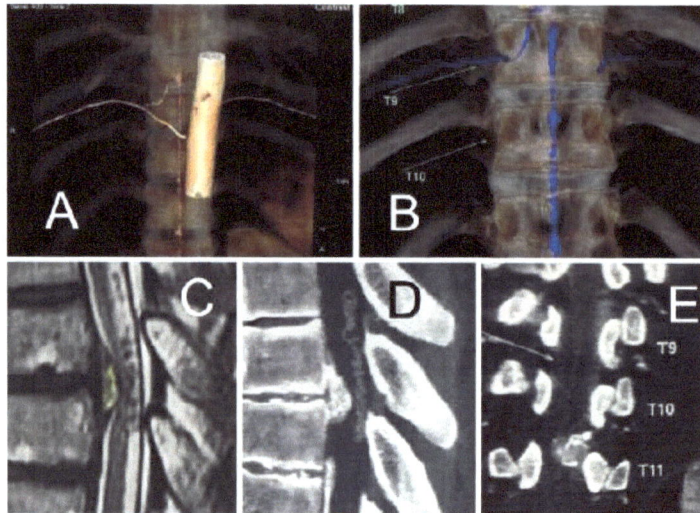

Fig. (2). (**a-b**) Display coronal CT angiography scans illustrating the foraminal entry level of the Magna radicular artery at T9-T10, (**b**) along with the presence of a medullary angioma, (c-e) at T10-T11. Electrocautery at the foraminal entry level of blood supply to the Adamkiewicz system should be avoided to prevent unintended spinal cord ischemia during the endoscopic procedure. The surgeon, in this case, opted to cancel the transforaminal endoscopic discectomy due to the heightened risk of spinal cord ischemia. Source: Reproduced under open access Creative Commons Attribution (CC BY) license (https://creativecommons.org/licenses/by/4.0/) from Vargas *et al*, 2023 [40].

There was a notable decline in the average preoperative Visual Analog Scale (VAS) score, which dropped from 8.53 ± 0.92 before surgery to 1.60 ± 2.06 post-surgery ($p < 0.0001$). This translates to an average VAS reduction of 6.93 ± 1.86. Out of the 15 participants, 14 (or 93.33%) witnessed a marked alleviation of their symptoms and reported better daily functionality. However, one individual displayed residual neurological impairments aligned with anterior spinal cord syndrome post-endoscopic discectomy. No cases of infection, unusual sensations, or numbness were noted, with the exception of one patient (referenced as patient #8 in Table **4**) who suffered paralysis. Subsequent to this incident, a postoperative CTA identified the AKA system in this patient. As a result of this complication, the authors updated their pre-surgical evaluation protocol for thoracic herniated discs to incorporate CTA as a key element (as depicted in Fig. **2**). Barring one patient, the CTA examinations for the other 14 participants of the study showcased clear visualization of the intercostal vessels, marking them from their genesis point on the descending aorta (illustrated in Fig. **3**).

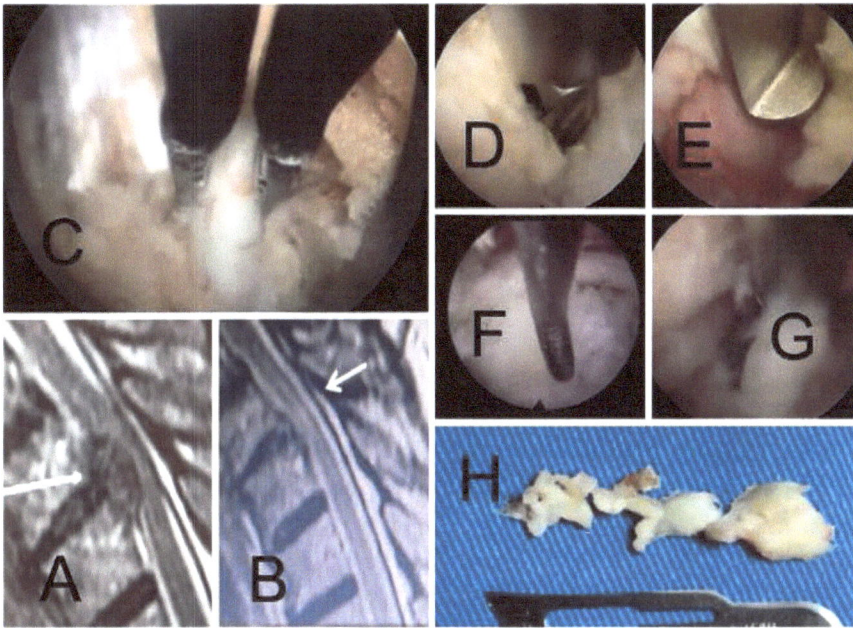

Fig. (3). Displays the preoperative (**a**) and postoperative (**b**) sagittal T2-weighted MRI scans of a patient who underwent transforaminal endoscopic T10/11 discectomy. The magna radicular artery was encountered (**c**) during the thoracic endoscopy, prompting the surgeon to perform a wide foraminoplasty utilizing an endoscopic drill (**d**) and Kerrison rongeur (**e**) to avoid electrocautery. The discectomy was then completed by using an endoscopic nerve hook (**f**) to deliver the herniation from beneath the posterior longitudinal ligament and removing it piecemeal with an endoscopic grasper (**g**) (**h**). Source: Reproduced under open access Creative Commons Attribution (CC BY) license (https://creativecommons.org/licenses/by/4.0/) from Vargas *et al*, 2023 [40].

Proposed AKA Classification

From the authors' clinical findings, we suggest categorizing patients set for thoracic discectomy into three classifications based on their painful pathology's proximity to the Adamkiewicz artery (AKA):

1. **Far-Type**: Here, the ailment is significantly separate from the AKA. Typical manifestations might include herniated discs, tumors, or vertebral fractures. For such patients, endoscopic decompression is a potential therapeutic route.

2. **Near-Type**: While the pathological condition isn't directly at the AKA's thoracic entry foramen, it's in the vicinity, perhaps at a neighboring level. The optimal surgical methodology for this category might be contested. Should surgery be essential, the pre-surgical strategy should focus on outlining measures to tackle AKA presence and mitigate spinal cord compression. Gentle and precise surgical handling is paramount, given the potential ischemic state stemming from the primary clinical syndrome. If there's ambiguity about achieving endoscopic

treatment without endangering the spinal cord further, opting for a broader laminectomy or an expanded costotransversectomy could be more suitable, as demonstrated in the authors' historical sequential case studies.

3. **Foraminal-Type**: The affliction is precisely at the Magna root artery's entry point. In such scenarios, both the nerve root and the Magna artery must remain intact, irrespective of the chosen surgical procedure. Considering the temporary use of an aneurysm clip on the intraforaminal Magna radicularis might be a viable choice in conventional surgeries or when feasible, especially if CTA findings are unclear. Temporary clipping of vessels powered by radicular arteries has been utilized when treating specific arteriovenous conditions in myelopathy-afflicted patients. Should there be no observable alteration in neurological assessments or any symptoms of lower limb heaviness in alert patients post-clipping, artery coagulation or ligation can be contemplated. In instances of fleeting weakness post-clipping, the clip can be detached, and blood pressure adjusted to prevent long-term impairments. Such a protocol aligns with recommendations in neurosurgery for particular fistulas and tumors. Nevertheless, for pragmatic reasons, these authors advocate for a comprehensive CTA, acknowledging that not all endoscopic spinal surgeons possess a neurosurgical background.

Example of AKA at the Surgical Level

When planning a thoracic endoscopic discectomy at the same surgical level as the Adamkiewicz artery's entry, thorough evaluation is paramount. Given the artery's role in supplying the anterior spinal cord, safeguarding it is vital to prevent ischemic issues and possible neurological impairments. Surgeons need to balance the benefits of the discectomy with the potential hazards to this artery. The authors' team encountered numerous patients requiring thoracic discectomy for spinal cord compression and myelopathy. However, in some cases, the surgical intervention was viewed as overly perilous, with a significant chance of paraplegia, leading to a preference for interventional care (Fig. **4**).

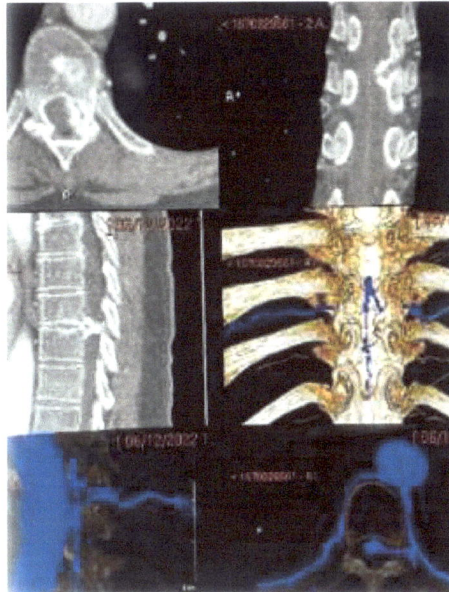

Fig. (4). Shown are CT and CTA scans of a 62-year-old myelopathic female referred for myelopathy symptoms for calcified T10/11 herniated disc with severe canal compromise.

For this particular case, the surgical extraction of the calcified thoracic disc herniation was considered too perilous. The entry of the AKA into the surgical neuroforamen raised concerns that it could be damaged during discectomy, especially given the need for spinal cord retraction and the presence of a sizeable calcified disc (Fig. **5**). After discussing the potential risks with the patient, the surgeon recommended a regimen of physical therapy focusing on gait and balance, along with spinal injections to address the intercostal nerve pain that initially led to seeking a spine specialist. Understanding the heightened risk of potential paraplegia from surgical intervention compared to non-surgical management, the patient concurred with the suggested approach.

DISCUSSION

Endoscopic spine surgery's adoption is expanding beyond the lumbar region, yet its application in the thoracic spine can jeopardize the spinal cord's vascular support, which is facilitated by three primary arteries. The anterior spinal artery nourishes the front two-thirds of the spinal cord, and the pair of posterolateral spinal arteries cater to its posterior third [26, 34]. The foremost vessel, the anterior spinal artery, emerges from the two vertebral arteries near the foramen magnum and is augmented by segmental medullary arteries from the aorta at each spinal tier [34]. The most prominent among these is the artery of Adamkiewicz or the arteria radicularis magna [4]. This artery can be traced to its source in the descending aorta, where 8 to 10 intercostal and lumbar arteries branch anteriorly and posteriorly [41]. The latter branches stem from the radiculomedullary artery and comprise muscular and dorsal somatic subdivisions. The radiculomedullary artery primarily divides into major anterior and minor posterior branches, with the artery of Adamkiewicz being the principal anterior radiculomedullary artery. As it approaches the intervertebral foramen, this artery usually lies close to, often in front of, the outgoing thoracic nerve and moves somewhat upwards and outwards along the spinal cord's front side [27]. In its upward course, the artery forms a distinctive "hairpin" curve, evident in angiograms, as it merges with the anterior spinal artery [7, 29, 42]. The comprehensive AKA process is illustrated in Fig. (5).

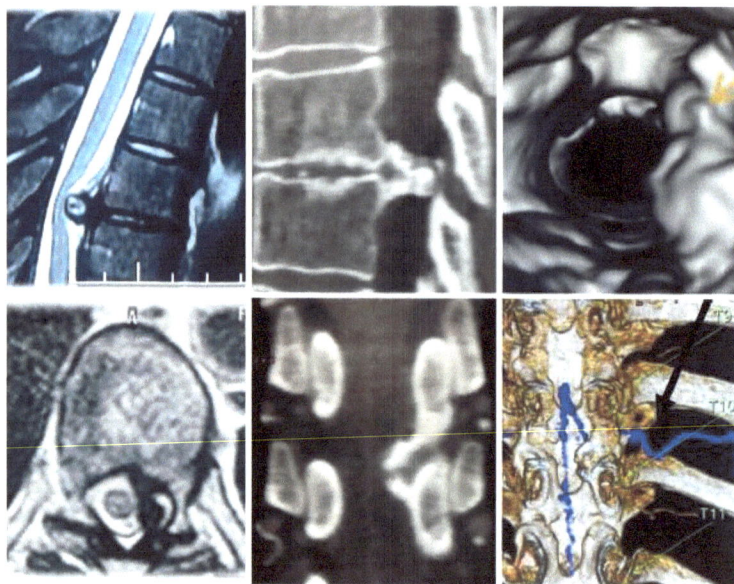

Fig. (5). MRI (left column), CT (middle column), and CTA (right column) scans of a 62-year-old myelopathic female referred for myelopathy symptoms for calcified T10/11 herniated disc with severe canal compromise. The canal compromise was substantial, and the AKA entered right underneath the disc herniation. Hence, discectomy carried a high risk of ischemic paraplegia. Non-surgical care with gait- and balance training and spinal injections were recommended.

Utilizing coagulation during transforaminal access for bleeding control and enhanced visualization comes with substantial risks. Recognizing the potential severe outcomes, the authors typically favor the slightly lateral interlaminar technique, offering direct access to the facet joint space. Yet, for patients displaying clear myelopathy due to a central calcified herniation with associated myelomalacia on thoracic MRI scans, the transforaminal method might be more apt. This approach specifically addresses calcified central herniations, a significant hurdle in thoracic spine endoscopy. The benefit of the transforaminal method is its reduced spinal cord manipulation since it focuses on the intervertebral disc beneath the dural sac. When the AKA system's position is verified *via* CTA, this technique can be a logical alternative to the interlaminar one, avoiding unnecessary coagulation of the foraminal root artery (Fig. **6**).

Fig. (6). Infogramm of the AKA protocol surgeons should employ when contemplating a thoracic discectomy.

CONCLUSION

The authors emphasize the importance of including a formal computed tomography angiography (CTA) in the preoperative diagnostic routine to clearly identify the Adamkiewicz system's entry into the thoracic spinal canal. This recommendation emerged from an unfortunate incident where a patient experienced postoperative paraplegia, deeply affecting everyone involved. The CTA protocols used in this study are well-established and widely applied [28, 33]. The efficacy of magnetic resonance angiography (MRA) in comparison to CTA for studying the Adamkiewicz system is under scrutiny [29]. As the Adamkiewicz artery might be missing in roughly 10% of patients [8], it is imperative for radiologists to meticulously trace the intercostal arteries during the arterial phase, which typically aligns with the radicular arteries' contrast filling [28]. Straying from this protocol could compromise the clear identification of the Adamkiewicz artery. The authors underline the significance of this methodology for endoscopic spinal surgery and other prevalent surgical treatments like infections, tumors, fractures, and deformities.

REFERENCES

[1]   Lin GX, Kotheeranurak V, Mahatthanatrakul A, *et al.* Worldwide research productivity in the field of full-endoscopic spine surgery: a bibliometric study. Eur Spine J 2020; 29(1): 153-60.
[http://dx.doi.org/10.1007/s00586-019-06171-2] [PMID: 31642995]

[2]   Lewandrowski KU, Soriano-Sánchez JA, Zhang X, *et al.* Surgeon motivation, and obstacles to the implementation of minimally invasive spinal surgery techniques. J Spine Surg 2020; 6(S1) (Suppl. 1): S249-59.
[http://dx.doi.org/10.21037/jss.2019.08.02] [PMID: 32195432]

[3]   Hofstetter CP, Ahn Y, Choi G, *et al.* AOSpine Consensus Paper on Nomenclature for Working-Channel Endoscopic Spinal Procedures. Global Spine J 2020; 10(2_suppl) (Suppl.): 111S-21S.
[http://dx.doi.org/10.1177/2192568219887364] [PMID: 32528794]

[4]   Li X, An B, Gao H, *et al.* Surgical results and prognostic factors following percutaneous full endoscopic posterior decompression for thoracic myelopathy caused by ossification of the ligamentum flavum. Sci Rep 2020; 10(1): 1305.
[http://dx.doi.org/10.1038/s41598-020-58198-x] [PMID: 31992790]

[5]   Ruetten S, Hahn P, Oezdemir S, Baraliakos X, Godolias G, Komp M. Operation of Soft or Calcified Thoracic Disc Herniations in the Full-Endoscopic Uniportal Extraforaminal Technique. Pain Physician 2018; 1(21;1): E331-40.
[http://dx.doi.org/10.36076/ppj.2018.4.E331] [PMID: 30045599]

[6]   Ruetten S, Hahn P, Oezdemir S, *et al.* Full-endoscopic uniportal decompression in disc herniations and stenosis of the thoracic spine using the interlaminar, extraforaminal, or transthoracic retropleural approach. J Neurosurg Spine 2018; 29(2): 157-68.
[http://dx.doi.org/10.3171/2017.12.SPINE171096] [PMID: 29856303]

[7]   N'da HA, Chenin L, Capel C, Havet E, Le Gars D, Peltier J. Microsurgical anatomy of the Adamkiewicz artery–anterior spinal artery junction. Surg Radiol Anat 2016; 38(5): 563-7.
[http://dx.doi.org/10.1007/s00276-015-1596-3] [PMID: 26627692]

[8]   Lindeire S, Hauser JM. Anatomy, Back, Artery Of Adamkiewicz. Treasure Island (FL): StatPearls 2022.
[PMID: 30422566]

[9]   Yeung A, Lewandrowski KU. Early and staged endoscopic management of common pain generators in the spine. J Spine Surg 2020; 6(S1) (Suppl. 1): S1-5.
[http://dx.doi.org/10.21037/jss.2019.09.03] [PMID: 32195407]

[10]   Lewandrowski KU, Yeung A. Lumbar Endoscopic Bony and Soft Tissue Decompression With the Hybridized Inside-Out Approach: A Review And Technical Note. Neurospine 2020; 17 (Suppl. 1): S34-43.
[http://dx.doi.org/10.14245/ns.2040160.080] [PMID: 32746516]

[11]   Lewandrowski KU, Yeung A. Meaningful outcome research to validate endoscopic treatment of common lumbar pain generators with durability analysis. J Spine Surg 2020; 6(S1) (Suppl. 1): S6-S13.
[http://dx.doi.org/10.21037/jss.2019.09.07] [PMID: 32195408]

[12]   Lewandrowski KU, De Carvalho PST, De Carvalho P Jr, Yeung A. Minimal Clinically Important Difference in Patient-Reported Outcome Measures with the Transforaminal Endoscopic Decompression for Lateral Recess and Foraminal Stenosis. Int J Spine Surg 2020; 14(2): 254-66.
[http://dx.doi.org/10.14444/7034] [PMID: 32355633]

[13]   Lewandrowski KU. The strategies behind "inside-out" and "outside-in" endoscopy of the lumbar spine: treating the pain generator. J Spine Surg 2020; 6(S1) (Suppl. 1): S35-9.
[http://dx.doi.org/10.21037/jss.2019.06.06] [PMID: 32195412]

[14]   Dowling Á, Lewandrowski KU, da Silva FHP, Araneda Parra JA, Portillo DM, Pineda Giménez YC. Patient selection protocols for endoscopic transforaminal, interlaminar, and translaminar decompression of lumbar spinal stenosis. J Spine Surg 2020; 6(S1) (Suppl. 1): S120-32.
[http://dx.doi.org/10.21037/jss.2019.11.07] [PMID: 32195421]

[15]   Gore S, Yeung A. The "inside out" transforaminal technique to treat lumbar spinal pain in an awake and aware patient under local anesthesia: results and a review of the literature. Int J Spine Surg 2014; 8: 28.
[http://dx.doi.org/10.14444/1028] [PMID: 25694940]

[16]   Yeung AT, Yeung CA. Minimally invasive techniques for the management of lumbar disc herniation. Orthop Clin North Am 2007; 38(3): 363-72.
[http://dx.doi.org/10.1016/j.ocl.2007.04.005] [PMID: 17629984]

[17]   Knight MTN, Ellison DR, Goswami A, Hillier VF. Review of safety in endoscopic laser foraminoplasty for the management of back pain. J Clin Laser Med Surg 2001; 19(3): 147-57.
[http://dx.doi.org/10.1089/10445470152927982] [PMID: 11469307]

[18]   Wu X, Wang J, Xu Z, *et al.* Bi-Needle PELD with Intra-Discal Irrigation Technique for the Management of Lumbar Disc Herniation. Pain Physician 2022; 25(2): E309-17.
[PMID: 35322986]

[19]   Jasper GP, Francisco GM, Telfeian AE. Clinical success of transforaminal endoscopic discectomy with foraminotomy: A retrospective evaluation. Clin Neurol Neurosurg 2013; 115(10): 1961-5.
[http://dx.doi.org/10.1016/j.clineuro.2013.05.033] [PMID: 23835307]

[20]   Jasper GP, Francisco GM, Telfeian AE. A retrospective evaluation of the clinical success of transforaminal endoscopic discectomy with foraminotomy in geriatric patients. Pain Physician 2013; 16(3): 225-9.
[PMID: 23703409]

[21]   Jasper GP, Francisco GM, Telfeian A. Outpatient, awake, ultra-minimally invasive endoscopic treatment of lumbar disc herniations. R I Med J 2013; 97(6): 47-9.
[PMID: 24905375]

[22]   Jasper GP, Francisco GM, Telfeian AE. Transforaminal endoscopic discectomy with foraminoplasty for the treatment of spondylolisthesis. Pain Physician 2014; 17(6): E703-8.
[PMID: 25415785]

[23]   Telfeian AE, Jasper GP, Francisco GM. Transforaminal endoscopic treatment of lumbar radiculopathy after instrumented lumbar spine fusion. Pain Physician 2015; 2(18): 179-84.
[http://dx.doi.org/10.36076/ppj/2015.18.179] [PMID: 25794204]

[24]   Telfeian AE, Jasper GP, Oyelese AA, Gokaslan ZL. Technical considerations in transforaminal endoscopic spine surgery at the thoracolumbar junction: report of 3 cases. Neurosurg Focus 2016; 40(2): E9.
[http://dx.doi.org/10.3171/2015.10.FOCUS15372] [PMID: 26828890]

[25]   Lyders EM, Morris PP. A case of spinal cord infarction following lumbar transforaminal epidural steroid injection: MR imaging and angiographic findings. AJNR Am J Neuroradiol 2009; 30(9): 1691-3.
[http://dx.doi.org/10.3174/ajnr.A1567] [PMID: 19369604]

[26]   Klakeel M, Thompson J, Srinivasan R, Mcdonald F. Anterior spinal cord syndrome of unknown etiology. Proc Bayl Univ Med Cent 2015; 28(1): 85-7.
[http://dx.doi.org/10.1080/08998280.2015.11929201] [PMID: 25552812]

[27]   Yadav N, Pendharkar H, Kulkarni GB. Spinal Cord Infarction: Clinical and Radiological Features. J Stroke Cerebrovasc Dis 2018; 27(10): 2810-21.
[http://dx.doi.org/10.1016/j.jstrokecerebrovasdis.2018.06.008] [PMID: 30093205]

[28]   Guziński M, Bryl M, Ziemińska K, Wolny K, Sąsiadek M, Garcarek J. Detection of the

Adamkiewiczartery in computed tomography of the thorax and abdomen. Adv Clin Exp Med 2017; 26(1): 31-7.
[http://dx.doi.org/10.17219/acem/62788] [PMID: 28397429]

[29]   Yoshioka K, Niinuma H, Ehara S, Nakajima T, Nakamura M, Kawazoe K. MR angiography and CT angiography of the artery of Adamkiewicz: state of the art. Radiographics 2006; 26 (Suppl. 1): S63-73.
[http://dx.doi.org/10.1148/rg.26si065506] [PMID: 17050520]

[30]   Charles YP, Barbe B, Beaujeux R, Boujan F, Steib JP. Relevance of the anatomical location of the Adamkiewicz artery in spine surgery. Surg Radiol Anat 2011; 33(1): 3-9.
[http://dx.doi.org/10.1007/s00276-010-0654-0] [PMID: 20589376]

[31]   Griepp RB, Ergin MA, Galla JD, *et al.* Surgery for acquired heart disease looking for the artery of adamkiewicz: A quest to minimize paraplegia after operations for aneurysms of the descending thoracic and thoracoabdominal aorta. J Thorac Cardiovasc Surg 1996; 112(5): 1202-15.
[http://dx.doi.org/10.1016/S0022-5223(96)70133-2] [PMID: 8911316]

[32]   Nijenhuis RJ, Leiner T, Cornips EMJ, *et al.* Spinal cord feeding arteries at MR angiography for thoracoscopic spinal surgery: feasibility study and implications for surgical approach. Radiology 2004; 233(2): 541-7.
[http://dx.doi.org/10.1148/radiol.2331031672] [PMID: 15358852]

[33]   Theologis AA, Ramirez J, Diab M, Preoperative CT. Preoperative CT Angiography Informs Instrumentation in Anterior Spine Surgery for Idiopathic Scoliosis. J Am Acad Orthop Surg Glob Res Rev 2020; 4(4): e19.00123.
[http://dx.doi.org/10.5435/JAAOSGlobal-D-19-00123] [PMID: 32377614]

[34]   Bican O, Minagar A, Pruitt AA. The spinal cord: a review of functional neuroanatomy. Neurol Clin 2013; 31(1): 1-18.
[http://dx.doi.org/10.1016/j.ncl.2012.09.009] [PMID: 23186894]

[35]   Amato ACM, Parga Filho JR, Stolf NAG. Predictors of Adamkiewicz artery and anterior spinal artery detection through computerized tomographic angiography. SAGE Open Med 2017; 5
[http://dx.doi.org/10.1177/2050312117711599] [PMID: 28616230]

[36]   Ruetten S, Hahn P, Oezdemir S, Baraliakos X, Godolias G, Komp M. Decompression of the anterior thoracic spinal canal using a novel full□endoscopic uniportal transthoracic retropleural technique—an anatomical feasibility study in human cadavers. Clin Anat 2018; 31(5): 716-23.
[http://dx.doi.org/10.1002/ca.23075] [PMID: 29577428]

[37]   Yue JJ, Long W. Full Endoscopic Spinal Surgery Techniques: Advancements, Indications, and Outcomes. Int J Spine Surg 2015; 9: 17.
[http://dx.doi.org/10.14444/2017] [PMID: 26114086]

[38]   Yeung AT, Yeung CA. Advances in endoscopic disc and spine surgery: foraminal approach. Surg Technol Int 2003; 11: 255-63.
[PMID: 12931309]

[39]   Rubino F, Deutsch H, Pamoukian V, Zhu JF, King WA, Gagner M. Minimally invasive spine surgery: an animal model for endoscopic approach to the anterior cervical and upper thoracic spine. J Laparoendosc Adv Surg Tech A 2000; 10(6): 309-13.
[http://dx.doi.org/10.1089/lap.2000.10.309] [PMID: 11132909]

[40]   Vargas RA, De Olinveira EM, Moscatelli M, *et al.* Identification of the Magna Radicular Artery Entry Foramen and Adamkiewicz System: Patient Selection for Open *versus* Full-Endoscopic Thoracic Spinal Decompression Surgery. J Pers Med 2023; 13(2): 356.
[http://dx.doi.org/10.3390/jpm13020356] [PMID: 36836589]

[41]   Kroszczynski AC, Kohan K, Kurowski M, Olson TR, Downie SA. Intraforaminal location of thoracolumbar anterior medullary arteries. Pain Med 2013; 14(6): 808-12.
[http://dx.doi.org/10.1111/pme.12056] [PMID: 23438301]

[42]   Murthy NS, Maus TP, Behrns CL. Intraforaminal location of the great anterior radiculomedullary artery (artery of Adamkiewicz): a retrospective review. Pain Med 2010; 11(12): 1756-64.
[http://dx.doi.org/10.1111/j.1526-4637.2010.00948.x] [PMID: 21134118]

SUBJECT INDEX

A

Abnormalities, associated spinal 56
Acid 52, 53
  folic 53
  valproic 52
Advanced multi-slice helical CT imaging 96
Air pollution 52
Analgesic opioid therapy 79, 80
Anastomosis 105
Anesthesia 29, 31, 68, 73, 74, 130
  intramuscular 74
  local 31
Angiographic portrayals 137
Angiography, magnetic resonance 138, 155
Anterior 43, 45, 100, 101, 102, 103, 116
  cerebral arteries (ACA) 43, 100, 101
  ethmoidal arteries (AEA) 45
  isthmus 101, 102, 103
  plagiocephaly procedure 116
Anterior spinal 141, 143
  artery system 143
  cord syndrome 141, 143

B

Bilateral sphenoids 9
Biopsies, diagnostic 2
Bleeding(s) 118, 154
  control 154
  proportional 118
Blood 94, 110, 129, 131, 145
  accumulation 131
  disorders 145
  leaking 129
  loss 94, 110
Bony 45, 147, 149
  ethmoidectomy 45
  foraminal stenosis 147, 149
Bony defects 8, 39, 52
  contiguous 52
Brain 2, 53

malformations 53
tumors 2
Breathing airway 44
Bunionectomy 44

C

Caesarean section 60, 61, 67, 74, 76, 77
Calcified disc, sizeable 153
Carcinoma 86, 87, 88
  lung 87
  mammary 86
Carcinomatosis 88
Cardiac arrhythmia 131
Cardiovascular 128, 129
  complications 129
  status 128
Cephalalgia 30, 128, 130
Cerebellar 7, 29, 55
  contour 55
  infarctions 7
  tonsil 29
Cerebral 7, 93, 94, 131
  abscesses 7
  angiography 131
  arteries post-bifurcation 93
  hemosiderosis 94
Cerebral artery 40, 43, 81, 82, 85, 88, 93, 95, 97, 99, 100, 101, 102, 103, 106
  anterior 43, 97, 99, 100, 101, 106
  bifurcation 95
Cerebrospinal fluid 8, 17, 40, 81, 82, 85, 88
  rhinorrhea 8, 17
Cervical discomfort 128
Chromosomal disorders 51
Cisterna magna cisternography 31
Computed tomography (CT) 15, 17, 24, 31, 130, 138, 143, 144, 145, 146, 150, 153, 154, 155
  angiography (CTA) 138, 143, 144, 145, 146, 150, 154, 155
Computerized tomography scanner 90

www.ingramcontent.com/pod-product-compliance
Lightning Source LLC
Chambersburg PA
CBHW041701210326
41598CB00007B/494